Disease Prev
through Vector Control

Guidelines for relief organisations

Madeleine C. Thomson
Liverpool School of Tropical Medicine

Oxfam
UK and Ireland

Books for a Change
Charing Cross Road
L'don
6 | 3 | 96

Published by Oxfam (UK and Ireland), 274 Banbury Road, Oxford OX2 7DZ, UK.
Designed by Oxfam Design Department OX1699/PK/95
Printed by Oxfam Print Unit
Oxfam is a registered charity no. 202918.

Contents

Figures and tables

Acknowledgements

Very many people contributed to the production of this manual by sharing knowledge and ideas, supporting field work, and last, but not least, providing funds. I cannot list everyone but I thank them all.

In particular I would like to thank John Seaman (Save the Children: SCF) for suggesting, and finding the initial funds for, the project. The Wellcome Trust, ICI, and the Jane Clayton Trust provided funds for field work in Pakistan, Ethiopia, and Malawi where I was kindly hosted by SCF staff. I would like to express my appreciation for all those working with SCF, Médecins sans Frontières (Holland), Action Aid, and other NGOs, as well as UNHCR, and the National Malaria/Vector Control programmes who helped me to gain an insider view of the refugee situations that they were dealing with. In particular I would like to thank Mennor Bouma and Julia Stucky. My visit to Geneva and WHO, UNHCR, and ICRC was also extremely valuable and I would like to thank those who took the time to discuss this subject with me.

Martin Birley and Bill MacDonald at the Liverpool School helped to establish the project, and many colleagues from Liverpool and London have helped with suggestions and corrections to the manuscript, including Dick Ashford, Guy Barnish, Des Chevasse, Stephen Connor, Chris Curtis, Pat Diskett, Sylvia Meek, Mike Service, and David Smith.

John Maunder (Medical Entomology Centre, Cambridge), Graham Mathews (IPARC), and Graham White (Zeneca) also improved the manuscript with their advice and ideas.

The final result is, however, my own responsibility. I am keen to hear from readers as to how useful they found the manual and their ideas for updating it for any future edition.

Madeleine Thomson
Liverpool January 1995

1 Vector-borne diseases and refugees

1.1 Introduction

1.1.1 Refugee[1] populations

Today more than 20 million refugees in countries throughout the world are dependent on international relief assistance. This number has risen dramatically over the last ten years, particularly in Africa, and, sadly, is likely to continue to do so. In addition to refugees, there are large numbers of internally displaced persons in countries such as former Yugoslavia, Rwanda, Afghanistan, Sudan, Ethiopia, Cambodia and Iran. There are over a million displaced people in Central America.

At least 80 per cent of registered refugees and displaced people are living in tropical or semi-tropical countries where vector-borne diseases, such as malaria, dengue, kala azar and sleeping sickness, are common and can have a high case-fatality rate if left untreated.

Outline of this book
The intention of producing these guidelines is to provide refugee relief workers with an overview of the problems associated with vector-borne diseases that they are likely to encounter, and a range of strategies for dealing with them. The type of information required for decision making on vector-control activities is described in section 1, and examples given of the management structures needed for an effective campaign. The major vector-borne diseases

---

1: The term 'refugee' is strictly defined by international law. It is used throughout these guidelines in a wider sense to include those fleeing from both war and famine, as well as those displaced within their own country.

and methods for their control are described in section 2. Section 3 presents community-based strategies for vector control. The choice and safe handling of insecticides is outlined in Section 4; and the final section gives recommendations for selection of spraying equipment. In the appendices there is a list of recommended texts; training courses; sources of advice; and the addresses of manufacturers of insecticide, spray machinery, bednets, and insect monitoring equipment.

These guidelines are not meant to be comprehensive but should be a good starting point for those interested in developing and strengthening preventive health-care programmes in refugee camps.

1.1.2 Vector[2]-borne diseases in refugee camps

Vector-borne diseases may be exacerbated in refugee populations for a number of reasons. In recent years *falciparum* malaria has been a serious cause of mortality in refugee camps on the Thai-Kampuchean border, in Pakistan, and currently in the Rwandan refugee camps in Zaire. It is particulary dangerous when refugees who have not been exposed to the disease before, and therefore have a low level of immunity, are forced to flee into a malarious area (for example, refugees from mountainous regions who flee into malarious lowland areas). Young children and pregnant women are particularly vulnerable to malaria and can suffer very high mortality as a result of infection.

Other vector-borne diseases that affect refugee populations occur as a result of crowded and unhygienic conditions. In recent years louse-borne typhus and relapsing fever have been found in refugee camps in Somalia and Sudan. Louse-borne diseases are not confined to underdeveloped countries, and louse-borne typhus was a major killer of POWs and concentration camp inmates in Europe during World War II. Louse-borne diseases are currently a major concern to health workers in former Yugoslavia.

There are several reasons why vector-borne diseases may represent serious threats to the health of refugee populations:

1 Refugees may lack immunity to a disease or the particular strain of the disease in the settlement area (e.g. malaria).
2 Refugees may have fled through an area infested with certain insect vectors (e.g. tsetse-flies — the vectors of human and cattle trypanosomiasis; sandflies — the vectors of kala azar).

2: In these guidelines the term 'vector' is given to any insect, tick, mite or rodent which transmits (carries) an infection from one animal or human host to another.

9

3 Refugees may have settled on land uninhabited by the local population because of insect vectors (e.g. blackflies, the vectors of river blindness).

4 Refugees may have lost their live-stock (in which case insects which normally bite both humans and animals will feed more on humans).

5 Refugees may live in unhygienic and crowded camps where certain vector populations may dramatically increase. Shortages of water may exacerbate this (e.g. body lice, the vectors of louse-borne typhus and relapsing fever and filth flies which transmit diarrhoeal diseases and trachoma).

6 Stress resulting from flight, fear and loss may exacerbate disease morbidity (e.g. malaria) and may be part of a nutrition-infection-malnutrition cycle. Refugees may have suffered minor or major trauma resulting in blood loss, or be infected with intestinal parasites. The resulting anaemia may make malaria infection life threatening

7 Such problems may be compounded by the breakdown of national vector control programmes in the areas from which the refugees have fled and in the host country. In the host country local resources may be overwhelmed by a sudden influx of refugees.

Vector control and public health measures

Prevention of vector-borne diseases through public health measures in a refugee setting may be more effective in reducing overall morbidity and mortality than curative care. However, all vector control programmes must be seen in the broader context of curative care, immunisation, and diagnostic facilities. Organisations interested in refugee health care should be aware of the risks of vector-borne epidemics, and prepare appropriate control strategies.

1.1.3 Definition of insect pests and vectors

Technical note: By scientific convention all creatures are identified by two names. The first (which always starts with a capital letter) is the 'genus' and the second the 'species' (e.g. *Homo sapiens* for humans). These specific namés are written in italics and are frequently abbreviated with just the first letter of the genus being given (e.g for the mosquito *Anopheles gambiae* the abbreviated version is *A. gambiae*).

In order to carry out a control programme against disease vectors it is important to distinguish between those insects, mites, ticks and rats that are merely a nuisance, and those that are mechanical and/or biological vectors. Control programmes are of two kinds: those aimed at reducing a pest population and those aimed at reducing the likelihood of disease transmission. Since some disease vectors are also serious pests, these two categories may overlap.

Nuisance pests

It is their presence in large numbers that defines a pest population as a nuisance. Control measures are generally designed to reduce the pest population or reduce the pest-human contact.

Mechanical vectors

These vectors transmit pathogens by transporting them on their feet or mouthparts. A good example is the housefly that may carry worms, eggs or bacteria from faeces to food-stuffs on its feet and, in this way, transmit diarrhoeal diseases. Mechanical vectors are usually only one of several transmission routes (diarrhoeal diseases are commonly transmitted where there is poor hygiene). Control measures can be designed to reduce the vector population, and to reduce the likelihood of disease transmission, for example, by covering food stuffs.

Biological vectors

These vectors are intrinsically involved in the life-cycle of the parasite or arbovirus (a virus transmitted by an arthropod vector), which must pass through the vector in order to mature to an infective stage capable of being transmitted to its human host. The parasites or arboviruses are acquired from, and are transmitted to, a human or animal host when the vector takes a blood meal. Mosquito vectors are always female since the female mosquito requires a blood meal to mature her developing eggs. In the case of malaria, the parasite usually takes about ten days to mature in the body of the mosquito vector before it is ready to infect a new host. Thus only older female mosquitoes are capable of transmitting malaria.

Because of this, control strategies against malaria vectors can either be designed to reduce the overall population of the vector species, or to reduce the likelihood of the average female mosquito living long enough to transmit the disease.

Both males and females of several other biological vectors, such as tsetse, mites, ticks, and fleas, can transmit diseases, since both sexes feed on host blood. Biological vectors may be a serious threat to health even when their numbers are relatively low.

1.1.4 Factors to be considered in vector-borne disease control

Many different kinds of information will be needed before decisions are made about the need for vector control in a refugee camp: information about the disease problem, about the refugee society, about financial and other resources available, and about the wider implications of vector-borne disease control in relation to the host community. Some of the factors to be considered are outlined below.

Diagnosis and epidemiological data

In many refugee situations the diagnostic facilities are very limited. Information about the most likely causes of 'fever of unknown origin' (including vector-borne disease) should be sought from epidemiological data and clinical symptoms. The setting up of a field laboratory and, in particular, the training of microscopists, are vital components of an effective control programme.

Data should be collected on:

• Who is infected? (adults, children, males, females, new arrivals, old residents). This information may show whether or not transmission is occurring inside the camp.

• Where do the infected people live or work? If the disease is localised, the control programme can be localised too, so that the control effort has the maximum effect.

The importance of training people to evaluate simple epidemiological data is shown in the following case studies: (from M. MacDonald, an entomologist, with UNBRO)

'...last August (1989) there was a frantic call from Site B that we must blast the camp with insecticides. The number of malaria cases seen at the hospital suddenly jumped from less than 100/month to over 500. But when we got up there and looked at the records we saw that all but two dozen were young adult males. It was obvious that there was not an outbreak of malaria within the camp

(In Sok Sann camp a number of children were shown to have malaria)....

when we ....plotted the distribution of P.falciparum cases in children under 14 we saw that there was a concentration in two sections of the camp. We made sure these sections were well covered with DDT spraying and did some night time barrier spraying with Deltacide and the cases amongst the children dropped.'

Identification and monitoring of vectors

An overall view of the likely pests and vectors to be found should be made on the basis of the known geographic distribution and ecology of the vectors. Within the camp environs, some vector species can be identified using simple reference texts or, if possible, with the help of a vector specialist.

Once the vector has been identified, it should be carefully monitored. *Pests* are easy to monitor, as their nuisance value is directly proportional to their numbers. *Vector species* may produce considerable levels of disease even when in relatively low numbers. Monitoring of vector populations by catching the insects when they come to bite people, or when they are resting, or by using some form of trap, will provide essential data on the locality of transmission: for example, are people being bitten while they sleep? Provision should be made for purchasing monitoring equipment. The population levels of certain vector species are closely associated with local climatic changes: rainfall, temperature, and humidity. Rainfall data in particular can be useful in predicting increases in vector populations.

Control strategy in a crisis
The level of response will depend on the seriousness of the situation. Does the epidemic cause a high mortality or morbidity when compared with other health problems? Many vector control programmes in refugee camps are introduced in response to a crisis. Being prepared for such eventualities will make the response much more effective.

By waiting for a crisis to occur before planning a control programme a delay is inevitable and makes it more likely that unsuitable insecticides will be used, because they are the only ones available. Items ordered from overseas may be delayed in customs for long periods. Spare parts for application machinery may take months to arrive and so a selection should always be bought at the time the machine is purchased.

In many cases where vector-borne diseases become a problem there is a 'let us spray everything' mentality. Spray programmes should always be regarded as an adjunct to other control methods (health education, sanitation, environmental health, biological control methods); although, in acute situations, a spraying programme can be initiated prior to any other control activity. Such a programme may be effective in the short term but is unlikely to be successful in the medium to longer term unless other control measures are also utilised.

Sociological factors and public education
While spraying might be a vital component in an emergency, there are important questions to be asked *before* commencing a control programme. Besides the epidemiological data to determine who is affected, there are sociological factors which need to be taken into consideration at the planning stage. Different cultural habits (such as purdah), and economic factors

(availability of cash income) will affect the outcome of a control programme. For example, insecticide treatment of women for lice control may be resisted; bednets may be exchanged for other items regarded as 'more valuable' by the refugees.

Public health education is a major tool in controlling vector-borne disease but is often neglected until a control programme has failed. All vector control programmes require at least the passive if not the active support and involvement of the refugees themselves. Residual spraying of insecticide in dwellings may be refused or washed off if the public are not informed and motivated. Informing refugees about vector-borne diseases, and training them in vector control, can also contribute to health care in the future. Providing information on the hazards of insecticides is also important.

Cost of control programme and choice of insecticide
Control programmes are rarely cheap, although they may be more cost effective than expensive curative programmes. Quality equipment and insecticides bought from well-known firms may be more expensive in the short term but they are recommended because in the long run they are cost-effective and safer.

The choice of insecticides will be determined by various factors: ability to kill the target insect; availability and registration in the country; formulation for particular application method; safety to humans and the environment; and cost.

The use of inappropriate insecticides is not only wasteful of precious resources but may be hazardous too.

Monitoring of programme
When a control programme is introduced, arrangements should be made to monitor its effectiveness. Poor coverage and application practices are two of the main reasons for the failure of control programmes. Many NGO's have a very short 'organisational memory'. Careful monitoring of a vector control programme will enable costly mistakes to be rectified and future programmes to be justified.

Justifying vector control programmes
The quality of health care in a refugee settlement is often superior to that provided to nationals in the host country. This may result in resentment on the part of local residents towards the refugees, and may also undermine the national health infrastructure.

The problems associated with providing refugee populations with health care facilities that are unavailable to the national population have been pointed out by Meek (1989):
'Control of malaria in sub-Saharan Africa is different from south-east Asia in that the frequency of infective bites per person is in many places so high that drastic reductions in mosquito populations would be needed to have any effect at all. Furthermore, very little malaria control is carried out in many African countries because of lack of resources and logistical capacity. It is, therefore, difficult to justify measures in a refugee camp which are not available in the host country, unless the incidence in the camps can be shown to be higher.'

NGO's working in such situations need to take these wider political considerations into account when deciding on a strategy for health care. There are several good reasons which can be put forward to the host community, to justify setting up a vector control programme:

1 Control is part of the national health strategy in the host country.
2 The refugee vector control programme is to be extended to the host community.
3 The level of disease in the refugee community is greater than that in the host community.
4 There is a risk of epidemics.
5 Disease or drug resistance may spread from the refugee community to the host community.
6 Disease or drug resistance may spread from the refugee community to their home community on repatriation.

1.2 Decision making in vector control

1.2.1 The basis of decision making

The vector-borne diseases found in refugee settlements will include those found in the local population as well as those generated by the unhygienic and overcrowded conditions that may be found within the camp. A number of key questions should be asked when deciding to undertake a vector control programme in a refugee camp:

• Is the vector-borne disease important in relation to other health problems?
• Is the disease being transmitted in or around the camp?

• Are vector control measures likely to have an effect?
If the answers to the last two questions is 'yes', then the next question is:
• What is the most efficient control strategy to adopt?

Relative priority
The relative priority of the vector-borne disease will depend on the threat of morbidity and mortality. Camps set up during an emergency for refugee or displaced people are characterised by two main phases:
The acute phase: this usually lasts 1-12 months depending on the initial health status of the refugees and the effectiveness of the relief organisation.
The chronic phase: the morbidity and mortality experienced by the refugees may be similar to that of the local population, depending on availability of basic services, degree of crowding, etc.

In some recent refugee emergencies the overall mortality in the acute phase has been up to 60 times the normal rate; and this is based on what is 'normal' in some of the world's poorest countries, where child survival is already extremely low. In the acute phase the importance of vector control must be assessed in relation to all the other inputs needed to sustain life.

The vital inputs required during the acute phase of a refugee emergency are:
• water, sanitation and shelter
• food distribution and nutrition interventions
• immunisations
• basic curative care (including surgery in a war zone).
and, in certain situations, vector control.

Situations when vector control is a priority
In certain circumstances, when there is a high threat of mortality or severe morbidity from a vector-borne disease, then vector control will become a priority. Vector control is warranted during the acute phase of a refugee emergency if any of the following conditions apply:
1 If the actual or threatened mortality rate from the disease is high and transmission is likely to occur in the camp; for example, where a large proportion of non-immune refugees are arriving in a camp where *falciparum* malaria transmission is likely to occur.
2 If the threatened mortality from the disease is high, the conditions exist for an epidemic, and the control is relatively simple. For example, louse-borne diseases are likely to reach epidemic proportions months after the setting up of a camp but mass delousing campaigns at reception centres and while

registering can greatly reduce the threat of an epidemic.

3 If there is a vector-borne epidemic in the locality which can result in a high mortality rate; for example, if there is a dengue haemorrhagic fever epidemic within the country and there is a likelihood of it spreading to the camp).

In the chronic phase, the need for vector control should be decided on the basis of the threat of morbidity, mortality, and the nuisance value of the particular insect.

Threat of morbidity and mortality

The main factors affecting the mortality rate caused by a vector-borne disease are:

• immune status of the population (i.e. proportion of non-immunes, under fives, pregnant women)
• current health status of the population
⋆ virulence of the parasite or virus
• availability and effectiveness of curative treatment.

The importance of vector control will depend on what other preventative and curative measures are available. The threat of mortality and morbidity from vector-borne diseases, and the methods for prevention and treatment are shown in Table 1.

Transmission

If the disease is not being transmitted within the camp then vector control efforts will be ineffective. Some diseases have a long incubation period. In a moving population it can be hard to tell where the infection was picked up. Immediate information should be sought on whether the vector is present in or near the camp; and whether epidemiological information supports the theory that transmission is occurring in the camp. For example, useful questions would be:

• *Have the infected people, that have fallen sick while in the camp, been in the camp for longer than the incubation period of the disease?*

If the answer is 'yes', then the disease is being transmitted in the camp.

• *Is the infection limited to new arrivals, or those that spend considerable time outside of the camp (e.g. men who are also fighters)?*

If the answer is 'yes', then the disease is being transmitted *outside* the camp.

Training health and sanitation staff to use epidemiological data to aid their choice of strategy will greatly improve the efficacy of any control measure undertaken. However, epidemiological data should be treated with caution, as there may be gender differences in reporting sickness to clinics; women in particular may be unable or unwilling to make use of health services, and their illnesses may be under-reported.

Table 1 The threat of mortality and morbidity from vector-borne diseases

Vector	Disease		Mortality and morbidity if untreated	Prevention and treatment	Notes
mosquitoes	malaria	falciparum	often fatal to non-immunes	drug therapy (resistance); vector control; environmental management; residual spraying; bednets	non-immunes, children and pregnant women are extremely vulnerable. explosive epidemics can occur
		vivax	can be fatal		
		malariae	rarely fatal		
		ovale	rarely fatal		
	yellow fever		fatal in 80% of severe cases	vaccination; isolation under bednets; vector control	monkey is the natural reservoir. vaccination is primary form of prevention
	dengue		not fatal	isolation under bednets; vector control	affects mainly non-caucasian children under 12 years old; epidemics occur when non-immunes enter endemic area
	dengue HF		fatal in 10-20% of cases		
	Japanese enceph.litis		fatal in 0.5-60% of cases	vaccination; isolation under bednets; vector control	transmitted from infected animals
	filariasis		not fatal – elephant-iasis (blocking of lymph ducts)	drug therapy; vector control	chronic disease which may is associated with poor, unsanitary, urban development
	other arboviral infections		not fatal	isolation under bednets; vector control	occasional occurrences or epidemics
lice	typhus		fatal in 10-40% of cases	antibiotics; change of clothing; delousing	characteristic of refugee populations crowded together in unhygienic conditions

18

Vector	Disease	Outcome	Treatment/control	Notes
filth flies	relapsing fever	fatal in 2-10% of cases	antibiotics; change of clothing; delousing	characteristic of refugee populations crowded together in unhygienic conditions
	trench fever	not fatal	antibiotics; change of clothing; delousing	characteristic of refugee populations crowded together in unhygienic conditions
	diarrhoeal disease	primary killer of under 5's	oral rehydration; antibiotics; hygiene/sanitation; vector control	may be an important transmission route
	eye disease (trachoma)	not fatal – severe eye impairment including blindness	antibiotics; hygiene/sanitation; vector control	may be an important transmission route
tsetse flies	Gambian sleeping sickness	death after years of infection	drug therapy (risky); vector control	sporadic human disease
	Rhodesian sleeping sickness	death within weeks of infection	drug therapy (risky); vector control	cattle trypanosomiasis (*nagana*) very important disease of cattle in Africa; human disease sporadic with occasional epidemics
sandflies	sandfly fever	not fatal	vector control	similar to about 80 other arboviral fevers transmitted by mosquitoes, sandflies, ticks.

Vector	Disease	Mortality and morbidity	Prevention and treatment	Notes
	cutaneous leishmaniasis	not fatal: severe skin lesions	drug therapy; vector control	may be epidemic in populations displaced into areas where animal reservoirs are common but may also be transmitted directly between humans.
	visceral leishmaniasis	fatal in 100% of cases	drug therapy; vector control	as above; epidemics are associated with social dislocation due to war/famine.
blackflies	onchocerciasis (river blindness)	not fatal – visual impairment, itchy skin, veru debilitating	drug therapy; vector control	blindness is more common in the savannah areas of West Africa than in the forest areas.
ticks	Crimean Congo HF	fatal in 2-50% of cases mild form Central Africa severe form Central Asia		transmission usually localised.
mites	typhus	fatal in 1-60% of cases depending on strain	antibiotics; repellents; insecti-cide impregnated; clothing	transmission usually localised – affects those who work in the bush (agriculturalists, military, hunters)
triatomine bugs	chagas disease	not immediately fatal; chronic debility	bednets; vector control	disease associated with poor housing
fleas	murine typhus	fatal in 2% of cases	antibiotics; vector control	occurs in unhygienic conditions with a large rat population
	plague bubonic pneumonic	fatal in 60% of cases fatal in 100% of cases within 48 hours	strict isolation; antibiotics; vector control	occurs in unhygienic conditions where there is a large rat population

In many situations it may be extremely difficult to determine where transmission is occurring. It may be necessary to maximise the use of minimal data. The scale of the control programme required to reduce transmission of a particular disease will depend on the dispersal range of the vector. A list of useful references on the epidemiology of vector-borne diseases is given at the end of this book.

1.3 Organisation of a control programme

Control programmes vary greatly in their complexity and effectiveness. Successful vector control programmes depend on well-informed, properly co-ordinated activities of a large enough control team, using appropriate and efficient control methods. Essential to such a programme is proper supervision to ensure that the measures are being carried out correctly, and an operational evaluation of the control methods to make sure that the objectives have been achieved.

1.3.1 Matching a control strategy to available resources
There are often a number of different strategies that might be adopted to control a particular vector. In the case of malaria, for example, possible strategies might include: destroying mosquito breeding sites; residual spraying with insecticide; or the provision of insecticide-treated bednets. Cost-benefit analysis can help in deciding which is the most appropriate method. This involves assessing and then comparing the effectiveness and the cost of differing control strategies. The purpose is to identify how to arrive at a specified objective at least cost; in other words, how to achieve the best results within a given budget. A guideline to this approach has been prepared by the WHO/FAO/UNEP/UNCHS Panel of Experts on Environmental Management for Vector Control: Phillips, M, Mills, A, and Dye, C (1993) *Guidelines for cost effectiveness analysis of vector control.*

The role of the host government
The largest refugee populations in the world today are in countries where the annual expenditure on health is extremely low. In these countries, national vector control programmes are rare, and, if they exist, usually face a permanent shortage of qualified personnel, transport, and funds. The appropriate government ministry should be consulted prior to the setting up of a control programme (particularly if it involves the use of insecticides). However, the

contribution that a ministry can make to the control programme will vary according to its own technical capacity at the time of the disease outbreak. During an epidemic, government resources may be over-stretched in protecting their nationals from the disease, and in such circumstances, NGOs may play an extremely important role. In a situation where the population has been displaced as a result of civil war it may not be possible to gain the support of the national government for a control programme.

National vector control programmes are often structured as vertical, single disease, control programmes (such as a National Malaria Control Programme). The advantage of vertical programmes in vector control is that the timing of an intervention (such as a spraying campaign) is often crucial; and vertical programmes may have more flexibility in ensuring a rapid response than a primary health care approach would have.

The role of International Organisations (IOs)

The Emergency Technical Cooperation Unit of the World Health Organisation (WHO) is committed to assist in emergency relief, including vector control, and may be able to procure, at short notice, insecticides, spraying equipment, protective clothing, and sanitation equipment. Expert advice and short-term consultations may be provided by WHO if requested through the Ministry of Health of the host government. Other international organisations with experience in vector control include the United Nations High Commission for Refugees and the International Commission of the Red Cross (ICRC).

The role of NGOs

The role of an NGO in a vector control programme will vary according to the particular situation and the level of involvement of the NGO in the overall running of health facilities within the refugee camp. NGO staff must make sure that they are aware of any national guidelines for vector control. The main areas of assistance that the NGO might provide are:

- access to technical expertise, by liaising with relevant IOs, government departments, academic or research institutions concerned with vector-borne diseases, and other NGOs; providing their own experienced personnel; employing consultant vector specialists; getting access to relevant international literature;
- funding of part or all of a vector control programme; in particular, funding for fuel, transport, salaries of spray personnel, insecticide, bednets, and equipment needed for environmental sanitation, such as spades, tractors, and garbage containers;

- running the vector control programme; in which case the NGO personnel must be aware of all aspects of vector control, including the need for planning and inter-sectoral collaboration.

The role of an entomologist (vector specialist)
The assistance of an entomologist (vector specialist) may be needed where vector control operations are being started. Local expertise should always be the first to be consulted. If national experts are not available then an expatriate consultant should be recruited. Organisations from which vector specialists might be recruited are listed in Appendix 1.

If a suitably qualified vector specialist is not available then a capable person, preferably a biologist, with the assistance of reliable reference texts and a hand-lens, should be able to identify the major pest groups. The texts listed in the references at the end of the book are useful in the identification of vector species.

The tasks of a vector specialist are:

1 **To predict the likely vector problems**. The advice of a vector specialist should be sought when a camp is being established, in order to reduce thelikelihood of siting the camp in a vector transmission zone, and to help to prepare control strategies in case the need arises.

2 **To identify the vector**. This may be particularly important in areas where there is no national vector control experience, and the specific mosquitoes responsible for malaria and viral diseases are not identified. In many areas of the world, the main vectors responsible for malaria have been identified, and their ecology and behaviour investigated.

3 **To locate the breeding sites of the vector**. This may be the most important function of a vector specialist, who will then be able to train other people in recognising vector habitats.

4 **To test insecticide susceptibility**. Insects can either be collected in the field and sent to a laboratory for testing or the tests may be undertaken by a skilled person under field conditions.

5 **To help to design the control programme** and train the vector control supervisors.

1.3.2 Evaluation and monitoring of vector control

Maps

A careful map of the refugee camp and its surrounding area (up to 2 km away if the security situation permits) at a scale of about 1:5000 should be made which shows all the individual sites which may be breeding grounds for insect vectors or rodent pests. A complete inventory of the type and location of all such sites should be made and used to provide a record of the time each site was inspected or treated.

> *An example of how breeding sites can be identified and controlled was given by an entomologist working in refugee camps in Sudan, who noted that mosquito breeding sites were localised, man-made and therefore easy to control: '(Several mosquito breeding areas were identified) .... in every case these were associated with the water supply (in particular the leaking water towers). ...the tukels closest to the tower were identified as one of the worst areas for cases of malaria in the settlement.' (C. Malcolm, Consultant Entomologist, UNHCR Eastern Sudan 1988)*

Recent advances in the use of satellite data make remotely sensed images a possible method for mapping uncharted areas. The Famine Early Warning System provides 'real time' satellite data which indicate the amount of plant growth in an area (which can alert authorities to potential famines). Rainfall data can be obtained from weather monitoring satellites, and high resolution images can be used for mapping.

Pest and vector surveys

Vector surveys are used to determine if insect or rodent pests and vectors are present. To do this the vector surveyor must be able to interpret signs of insect or rodent infestation and be able to identify which species are present. Monitoring should take place on a regular basis (once a week for larval mosquitoes) during the normal transmission season. Simple record sheets should be prepared on which to record the type of survey, the date, time, area, and the insects collected.

Surveys may involve active searches for insects and rodents, the use of bait or light traps, or the capture of insects attracted to feed on humans or animals. Such collections must be made regularly to monitor the abundance and type of vector or pest present. The addresses of manufacturers of insect traps are given in Appendix 2.

Since malaria mosquitoes usually bite at night, surveying adult mosquitoes in a refugee settlement is often made difficult by the lack of access to the camp at night to collect mosquitoes. Unless well trained and motivated refugees can be found to make such collections, insect traps, which can run with little supervision, or early morning spray collections, may be more appropriate.

Operational indicators
A simple list of operational indicators for a particular control programme should be made and kept up to date (see Table 2 for an example of operational indicators for malaria mosquito control).

Evaluation and monitoring of epidemiological information
Under the conditions prevailing in a refugee camp epidemiological information is best gathered by a small sample survey. This is often far more reliable than that emanating from a deficient universal coverage system; another advantage is that the results of a sample survey are rapidly available. Sample surveys may be based on records of hospitals, clinics, dispensaries. These data, even if biased by various factors, may indicate trends in the epidemiology of the disease. Most diseases vary seasonally, and samples should be carried out systematically throughout the transmission season. There are a number of reference texts which cover the procedures used to conduct epidemiological surveys and analyse their results, some of which are given in the references at the end of the book.

1.3.3 Training of the vector control team
The personnel required for a vector control team, and the level of training likely to be necessary are shown in Table 3.

On-the-spot training of sanitation workers and supervisors should be a regular and continuous feature of the vector control team. Even experienced workers should have annual refresher courses in control operations, public education, and insecticide safety. Such courses should be as practical as possible. Suitable written material and posters should be produced in the appropriate language.

Training manuals and course materials for senior and junior field staff should be obtained and adapted for local use. WHO produce a training manual for field staff working on a malaria control programme; another manual is provided for their tutor. GIFAP produce training material for users of agricultural pesticides which could be adapted for a vector control team. 'Home study' training courses

Table 2 Operational indicators for malaria mosquito control

Indoor residual spraying	Percentage of structures totally or partially covered in relation to target. Refusal rate, spot check of dosage and date of application of insecticide. Assessing and monitoring the susceptibility of vectors to insecticide.
Space spraying indoor and outdoor	Frequency and regularity of application. Coverage of applications. Timing of application. Assessing and monitoring the susceptibility of vectors to insecticide.
Larviciding operations	Assessing and monitoring the susceptibility of vector larvae to insecticide. Frequency, regularity and dosage of larviciding application. Estimated area covered and percentage of population protected. Regularity and coverage of entomological evaluation.
Environmental modification	Indication of the type and size of the operation, and the stage of development. Estimated percentage of population protected. Regularity and coverage of entomological monitoring.
Screening of houses	Percentage of dwellings screened. Degree of screening (partial or complete). Percentage of population protected.
Bednets, repellents	Random sampling survey to assess whether bednets or repellents are properly used. Frequency of use. Condition of bednets. Acceptability of repellents. Percentage of population protected. Percentage of most vulnerable groups protected.
Entomological laboratory and field	Percentage of trained field entomologists employed. Percentage of training undertaken. Number and frequency of entomological surveys undertaken in relation to plan

Table 3 Personnel required for vector control team

Personnel	Tasks	Training required
Public Health Officer/Chief Sanitarian/ Vector Control Officer	To assess vector problem, liaise with national and international experts if necessary, plan control programme, monitor control operation using entomological and operational indicators, train vector control supervisors, liaise with medical personnel and water engineer and instruct administrator.	Should already have training in public health including general vector control principles. If additional training is required then should attend national training course if available, inter-camp training course that may be set up or, if an expatriate, may attend short courses in vector control prior to arrival in country. Should have access to relevant literature and advice.
Administrator	To organise logistics of control programme, including employing sanitation/spray personnel, organising availability of transport, fuel, insecticide, shovels, camping equipment for field team if necessary, training programme of field staff.	Should be aware of importance of a particular vector problem, the need for timely interventions and the specifications for purchasing good quality bednets, insecticides, spray machinery. Should organise budget and account for moneys spent.
Supervisor	To inspect work, fill out operational indicator forms, identify current or potential vector breeding sites, Identify vector groups (such as anopheline mosquito larvae) train sanitation/spray personnel. One supervisor for every 6-10 sanitation/spray workers.	3-week training covering general theory of vector control, identification, of vector, breeding and resting sites, health education, training of sanitation workers, supervision, including filling in forms of operational evaluation, maintenance of spray machinery, safe use of insecticides.
Sanitation/ spray personnel	Draining swampy area, assisting in latrine building, residual spraying of insecticide. May be permanent or temporary staff.	3 days' practical training in control techniques, simple health education, safe use of insecticides. The methods of operational evaluation and supervision should be clearly explained.
Water engineer	Assistance with environmental sanitation, and the design and maintenance of water supply systems.	Should have access to relevant literature on vector control and to advice where necessary.
Medical personnel	Assess threat posed to refugee population by vector-borne disease and provide suitable epidemiological data from sample survey of refugee population. May liaise with Ministry of Health, national and international centres of expertise.	Should have familiarity with using health data to assess needs. Should have access to relevant literature and advice where necessary.

in entomology and epidemiology are available from the Centre for Disease Control (Atlanta, USA). These courses consist of a combination of lessons, manuals, outside reference material, and practical exercises, and proficiency and comprehension can be tested. CDC and WHO also produce a wide range of slide collections, covering a range of subjects related to vector-borne disease transmission and control, which can be used in training sessions for staff. A series of four-page technical briefings on health, water, and sanitation have been produced by the Intermediate Technology Centre.

Short courses may be available at certain institutes; such as the two-day louse and scabies eradication course run at the Medical Entomology Centre in Cambridge, or the course at the Liverpool School of Tropical Medicine course on community health in developing countries.

2 Major vector-borne diseases and their control

2.1 Introduction

This section does not provide a comprehensive list of all the vectors that might be encountered in a refugee settlement. The intention is to describe the most important vectors that may occur, and to give particular attention to those that may be controlled successfully within a camp setting. Table 4 gives information on different vector groups that is likely to determine the type of control programme that may be undertaken. Insects which have a short flight range, localised breeding or resting sites (for example, mosquitoes which rest inside buildings) will be the easiest to control. Wherever possible, local advice should be sought on the particular vector species that may be found in the environment of the camp.

The section is divided into sub-sections dealing with the diseases transmitted by specific vectors.

2.2 Mosquito-borne diseases

Mosquitoes are vectors of malaria, filariasis, and some arboviral infections. Female mosquitoes may feed on a variety of mammals, birds, and reptiles, each species having its own preferences for a particular source of blood. Many species of mosquitoes bite people, but only some of them are vectors of disease. Although all mosquitoes lay their eggs either in water or on the moist surfaces at the water's edge, each species has a particular ecological niche, and their breeding sites can be very specific. Control measures must be targeted to the specific mosquito species that is causing the problem.

Table 4 Generalised biological information on insect vectors that affect the feasibility of control

Insect vectors	Vector species	Disease	Breeding sites	Resting sites	Transmission	Blood source source	Dispersal range range	Control feasibility
mosquitoes	*Anopheles*	malaria; filariasis; arboviruses	swamps, still water, containers	indoors/ outdoors	night	people and animals	2 k	can be very effective – need specialist advice
	Aedes	encephalitis; filariasis	containers, small pools of stagnant water	indoors/ outdoors	day	people and animals	0.1 – 0.8km	can be very effective – need specialist advice
	Culex	filariasis; encephalitis	organically polluted water	indoors/ outdoors	day and night	people and animals	0.1 – 0.8km	can be very effective – need specialist advice
lice	*Pediculus*	typhus; relapsing fever; trench fever	clothing on human body or that has been worn within the last two weeks.	clothing on human body	day and night	people only	n/a	very effective and simple
filth flies	*Musca*	eye disease; diarrhoeal disease	organic matter, faeces, food, corpses	indoors/ outdoors	day	n/a	5km	sanitation very important

tsetse-flies	*Glossina*	sleeping sickness	soil	tree trunks	day	people and animals	2 – 4km	need specialist advice
sandflies	*Phlebotomus Lutzomia*	sandfly fever; leishmaniasis	mud cracks, termite hills, animal burrows, mud walls	indoors/ outdoors	night	people and animals	600m	need specialist advice
blackflies	*Simulium*	river blindness	fast-flowing rivers	outdoors	day	people and animals	10km	need specialist advice
ticks/mites	*Ixodidae Trombuciilidae*	typhus	vegetation	outdoors	day	people and animals	n/a	destroy vegetation
cone-nosed bugs	*Reduviidae*	chagas disease	cracks in walls and furniture	indoors	night	people and animals	10 -20m	insecticide control simple
fleas	*Xenopsylla*	plague; murine typhus	rats	with rats	night and day	people and animals	n/a	treat rat burrows with insecticide before controlling rats

31

Table 5 Mosquito groups and the diseases they transmit

Mosquito	Disease	Distribution
ANOPHELINE *Anopheles* (e.g.*A. gambiae* the main malaria vector in Africa)	malaria	endemic in most countries between latitude 30^0N and the Tropic of Capricorn in the south with northerly extensions in Turkey, Syria, Iraq, Iran, Afghanistan and China
	Bancroftian filariasis	endemic in tropical Africa, Middle East, South Asia, Far East and New Guinea, Tropical America
	Brugian filariasis	South-east Asia
	arboviral diseases	Africa
CULICINE *Culex* (e.g. *C.quinquefasciatus* the main vector of elephanti-asis in urban areas)	Bancroftian filariasis	endemic in tropical Africa, Middle East, South Asia, Far East and New Guinea, Tropical America
	Japanese encephalitis	Siberia, Japan, Korea, China, Indonesia, Singapore, Malaysia, Thailand, Vietnam, Burma, Nepal, India and Sri Lanka. Epidemics in Japan and Korea.
Mansonia major biting nuisance and occasional vector	Brugian filariasis	South-east Asia and South-west India
	arboviral diseases	Africa, Americas
Aedes (e.g. *A. aegypti*, the main vector of urban yellow fever and dengue)	yellow fever	endemic in West and Central Africa and in north and eastern parts of South America. Epidemics occur in central America.
	arboviral diseases - dengue haemorrhagic fever (DHF)	eEndemic throughout the tropics, particularly Asia, the Pacific and Caribbean. While dengue occurs in Africa DHF has not been recorded
	other arboviral disease	highly endemic in Africa and Asia and also found in the Americas
	Bancroftian filariasis	South Pacific, South Asia

Mosquito disease vectors are divided into to two groups, the *anophelines* and the *culicines*, which can be readily distinguished by characters that can be seen by the naked eye. Sanitation workers can be trained to recognise the different types of mosquitoes using the key in Appendix 3. Mosquito groups and the diseases they transmit are shown in Table 5, and Table 6 gives details of control methods which are available for different types of mosquito.

2.2.1 Malaria

Malaria is the most important vector-borne disease worldwide in terms of morbidity and mortality. It is considered by the major relief organisations to be one of the five top causes of child mortality in the acute phase of a majority of refugee emergencies. Its severity is often dependent on the level of immunity built up in an individual from previous exposure to different malaria parasite species and strains. The movement of refugees from one area to another often brings them into contact with malaria forms to which they have no immunity, which can result in epidemics of severe malaria developing. This might necessitate mass drug treatment plus vector control measures. Where women have a low level of acquired immunity, malaria is a major cause of maternal death, spontaneous abortion, stillbirth, and premature delivery. This is particularly true during a first pregnancy. All malaria is transmitted by *Anopheles* mosquitoes.

Anopheles mosquito: biological features
- most breed in still water
- breed in unpolluted water
- females feed in the evening or at night
- fly up to 2-3 km from breeding site
- only older females (2 weeks or more) can transmit malaria
- some insecticide resistance

Distribution: tropical and subtropical regions where water is available.

Characteristics: abundance can be highly seasonal and is linked to the timing and length of the rainy season. The population increases during the rainy season, when pools of water, representing potential breeding sites, are widespread.

Disease transmission: transmits four species of malaria (*ovale, malariae, vivax,* and *falciparum*). *Falciparum* malaria is the most important as it is particularly dangerous to those without acquired immunity. In any one area of the world malaria is mainly transmitted by one or two *Anopheles* species.

33

2.2.2 Control programmes

Control programmes are highly specific to the species of mosquito involved in transmission. If a national malaria programme is not being undertaken then specialist advice from an experienced entomologist will be needed to ascertain the likely effectiveness of a control programme.

Control options in an emergency situation will depend on the level of information and technical skill available. Assistance should be sought at once from national or international sources. Meanwhile, measures to reduce potential breeding sites should be started immediately. In Africa it can be assumed (until proved otherwise) that malaria vectors bite at night and rest indoors, and control measures can be taken accordingly (seeTable 6, p. 36).

2.2.3 Arboviral infections

The term 'arbovirus' is used to describe any virus transmitted by an arthropod (insect, mite or tick). There are over 400 arboviruses but only a hundred of these have been shown to cause clinical symptoms in humans. Those which cause major diseases are well studied, at least in some areas. These include dengue and dengue haemorrhagic fever, yellow fever, and Japanese encephalitis. Arboviral diseases all occur naturally in non-human hosts, such as monkeys or pigs. Most are transmitted from their animal host by a range of mosquitoes or ticks.

Dengue and yellow fever

Dengue and yellow fever are usually transmitted by *culicine* mosquitoes belonging to the *Aedes* genus.

Aedes: biological features
* 'container breeders'
* short flight range (30m)
* eggs can survive drying out (unlike *Anopheles*)
* most species bite and rest outdoors
* some insecticide resistance
* usually bite during the day.

Distribution: *Aedes aegypti* (the most common urban vector of arboviral diseases) is found widely throughout the tropics.

Characteristics: it breeds in water held in man-made containers, such as water storage jars, pots, tin cans, and old car tyres. It is nearly always associated with human habitats and mainly bites humans.

Disease transmission: dengue is endemic throughout the tropics but tends to occur in periodic epidemics. Dengue itself is fairly benign but it may be associated with dengue haemorrhagic fever or dengue shock syndrome, which are severe, often fatal diseases. Yellow fever, in its severe form, is also often fatal.

Control programmes: will vary according to the specific mosquito vector involved. Effective vaccines are available against yellow fever and these should be used as the first preventive measure. Control of *Aedes* vectors is practicable in an urban environment but is usually impossible in a forested area, where the mosquitoes breed in dispersed natural water pools in leaf axils or tree holes.

2.2.4 Filarial infections

Unlike malaria or arboviral infections that may be transmitted by a single bite of a single mosquito, filarial infections require repeated inoculations of the infective larvae, perhaps hundreds per year, before the worms are present in sufficient numbers to produce the symptoms of disease.

Bancroftian filariasis (elephantiasis)

This is caused by the parasitic worm *Wuchereria bancrofti*. The disease is widespread in the tropics, especially in urban environments, and is a chronic diseases that may take several years to manifest itself after infection.

Transmission: In rural areas Bancroftian filariasis is transmitted by the same vectors that transmit malaria and so is often controlled as a by-product of malaria control campaigns. In urban environments (and a refugee settlement can often be classified as urban even when it is in a rural area) the vector *Culex quinquefasciatus* is the most important vector.

Control programmes: these should be part of an overall improvement in community level sanitation. The building of non-fly proof latrines in urban areas has been shown to result in an increase in filariasis but this is only manifest after a number of years.

Brugian filariasis (elephantiasis)

This disease is caused by the parasitic worm *Brugia spp*. It is found in India and South Asia, predominantly in rural situations. It is a chronic diseases that may take several years to manifest itself after infection.

Transmission: usually transmitted by night-biting mosquitoes *Mansonia* spp.

Control programmes: the distribution and prevalence of the disease has been considerably reduced by the systematic removal of host plants from *Mansonia* larval breeding habitats.

Table 6 The choice of control method for different mosquitoes

Mosquito behaviour	Control programme	Vector species	Control of transmission	Control schedule
mosquito bites indoors	screening of windows, doors, eaves	*Anopheles* spp., *Culex* spp. few important *Aedes* spp. *Mansonia* spp.	immediate none or partial effectiveness	when house is built. Repair annually.
mosquito bites indoors at night	bednets	*Anopheles* spp. (no *Aedes* spp.) *Mansonia* spp. *Culex* spp.	immediate none or partial effectiveness	new bednet every 2-5 years
	insecticide impregnated bednets		partial or complete effectiveness	net impregnation every 6-12 months
mosquito rests indoors	indoor residual spraying	*Anopheles* spp, *Aedes aegypti* (no other *Aedes* spp.) *Culex* spp. *Mansonia* spp.	2-3 weeks partial or complete effectiveness	every 3-6 months, prior to transmission season
mosquito larvae attach to roots of aquatic vegetation (especially the water lettuce *Pistia stratiotes*)	removal of vegetation (especially water lettuce) from standing water	all *Mansonia* spp.	partial or complete effectiveness	check possible breeding sites weekly in the main growing season

(all mosquitoes)			
destruction of breeding sites	most vector species	2-3 weeks total effectiveness	permanent
larviciding	Anopheles, Culex, Mansonia, Aedes (except where breeding sites are unknown or inaccessible)	2-3 weeks partial/total effectiveness	every 2-3 weeks for Anopheles, every 2-3 months for Aedes
space spraying	Standard control method for Aedes simpsoni; effective against all other vector spp. but must be done at time when air conditions are right (early morning or in the evening)	must be undertaken daily until situation controlled. immediate, can be very effective	weekly after an attack phase of 10 days
repellents	all mosquitoes	immediate, lasts 1-6 hours; used during period of biting; very effective	daily during hours of biting

2.3 Fly-borne diseases

Filth flies which belong to the *Musca* genus can be important mechanical vectors of diarrhoeal diseases (most commonly the 'house fly' *Musca domestica*) and eye diseases (most commonly *Musca sorbens*).

Filth flies (Musca spp.): biological features
- breed in organic matter: garbage (*M. domestica*) and human faeces *(M. sorbens)*
- feed on food and organic matter (*M. domestica*) eye and wound secretions (*M. sorbens*)
- eight days from egg to adult at 35°C
- populations can increase very rapidly
- seasonal variation in abundance
- frequent insecticide resistance.

The other common filth flies — blue and greenbottles (*calliphona, lucillia* spp.) also breed in organic matter (including corpses), particularly in latrines, but may be much less important than the *Musca* group in disease transmission.

Distribution: worldwide

Characteristics: flies occur everywhere there is suitable breeding material, and the temperature and humidity are suitable for development. Fly numbers will increase with warmer weather, and very large numbers can build up under optimum conditions (i.e. <35°C and relative humidity of 50 per cent).

Disease transmission: flies transmit a number of different diseases mechanically but are never the sole transmission route (multiple transmission routes are the norm). It is usually impossible to tell how important fly transmission is in the occurrence of any disease that may be fly-borne.

2.3.1 Diarrhoeal disease

Diarrhoeal diseases, (such as shigella, salmonella, and cholera) are transmitted by houseflies (especially *M. domestica*). They can be a major killer of young children and therefore houseflies must be considered as a potential health hazard.

2.3.2 Eye disease

Flies which are attracted to the secretions around the eyes and to wounds (usually *M. sorbens*) may be particularly important in transmitting trachoma, a chronic disease of the eye that can lead to visual impairment, even blindness. The highest prevalence of trachoma has been recorded in Egypt and the Middle East. It was a major problem in the Somali refugee camps in 1980/81.

2.3.3 Control programmes

Control programmes for flies should, wherever possible, be based on providing suitable and effective methods of sanitation and garbage disposal. Hygienic disposal of rubbish in market areas may be a particularly important factor in disease control. Fly traps (such as sticky fly-papers) and poisoned baits may help to keep numbers down. These, combined with fly screening of rooms, should be a priority in communal kitchens, clinics, and feeding centres.

Adequate water supply for regular face washing is important in trachoma control, and water and soap for hand washing is essential for control of diarrhoeal diseases.

Insecticide control of flies is recommended when an epidemic of cholera, dysentery, or trachoma is threatened or underway. Preparations should be made in advance (including testing for insecticide resistance) so that fly numbers can rapidly be brought under control should the need arise. Fogging with a suitable insecticide can be an extremely effective way of reducing fly numbers if properly undertaken. It is, however, very expensive and usually needs to be repeated at weekly intervals.

2.3.4 Insecticide resistance

Filth flies are able to develop resistance to insecticides extremely rapidly. In many parts of the world they are resistant to organochlorines, organophosphates, and often pyrethroids. For this reason insecticide treatment for flies should only be undertaken if absolutely necessary, and bioassays should be conducted to test for insecticide resistance prior to any campaign. Residual spraying for fly control is not recommended since it is likely to enhance the development of resistance but, when undertaken for malaria control, may also have the effect of reducing housefly numbers.

Fly control in UNWRA camp: 'The source of the housefly problem was identified as possible insecticide resistance in the housefly population as well as increased breeding due to the destruction and disruption of sanitation services around the time of the Israeli invasion. The insecticide resistance was proved in laboratory tests at Porton Down with Lebanon-collected flies and alternative insecticides, to which the flies were still susceptible, were recommended. The need to avoid unnecessary routine insecticide use was stressed since the flies were resistant to all the major available insecticides except pyrethroids and resistance to this group could be expected to appear eventually if pyrethroids were used regularly.'

Harris (1990) Unpublished report from NRI

2.4 Louse-borne diseases

Body lice may be widespread in impoverished communities in temperate climates or in mountainous areas in tropical countries (or where nights are cold). They are the only known vector of louse-borne epidemic typhus and relapsing fever. These diseases may be rife in refugee camps, POW camps, and prisons and can be fatal if untreated.

Body lice (Pediculus humanus humanus) : biological features
- spend entire life on human clothing — not on head
- adults and nymphs soon die if not on host (2 hours — 2 days)
- egg hatching time 4-7 days
- some insecticide resistance

Table 7 Lice as vectors of disease

Lice	Disease	Distribution
body lice (*Pediculus humanus humanus*)	louse-borne typhus (*Rickettsia prowazeki*) (symptomless carriers exist among older age groups throughout the world including Europe)	recent epidemics have occurred in mountainous areas in East and Central Africa and in some high Andes communities in South America
	louse-borne relapsing fever (*Borrelia recurrentis*)	recent occurrences in the Ethiopian region, Somalia and Sudan; its incidence in the world and Africa in particular, is increasing
	trench fever (*Rochalimaea quintana*)	found occasionally in Central America and Europe
head lice (*Pediculus humanus capitis*)	not a disease vector but may produce allergies which result in 'lousiness'	worldwide
pubic ('crab') lice (*Pthirus pubis*)	not a disease vector but often associated with sexually transmitted diseases	worldwide

Distribution: worldwide.

Characteristics: body lice live in clothing (eggs and nymphs are mainly in inaccessible seams and corners). They feed regularly on their human host. They cannot be transferred to another host without direct and prolonged contact between the clothing of individuals. They can only survive for about a week off the host and then only as eggs.

Disease transmission: louse-borne diseases occur where lice numbers per individual are high and where lice are readily transmitted between individuals; e.g where people are crowded together, with insufficient clothing in cold conditions and where washing facilities are lacking (lice transfer is most likely from a feverish person or a corpse).

2.4.1 Louse-borne typhus

This disease is transmitted solely by faeces of contaminated lice through skin abrasions; or through mucous membrane by inhalation. The faeces are infective for three months. Non-lousy persons who come into contact with louse faeces are likely to be infected.

2.4.2 Louse-borne relapsing fever

This disease is transmitted when infective lice are crushed and the contents rubbed into abrasions or mucous membrane (common when people crush lice between finger nails or teeth). Infection of non-lousy persons is unlikely.

2.4.3 Trench fever

This disease is very rare, and not fatal.

2.4.4 Control programmes

These should be based on mass delousing, particularly when refugees arrive at camps, if they are carrying large numbers of body lice. Because of the severe threat of mortality from louse-borne typhus and relapsing fever, louse control programmes should be initiated immediately, whenever and wherever there is a threat of louse-borne disease.

De-lousing should be done at the main reception centre or where people are being admitted to hospitals or feeding centres. Equipment should include a steam, boil or dry heating facility, clean clothes to be worn while contaminated clothes are being treated, and a drying area.

Heating treatment may use up large amounts of scarce fuel. It might be possible to construct a fuel-efficient steaming barrel (Fig. 1). Solar heating systems should be investigated.

Fig 1 Steaming barrel

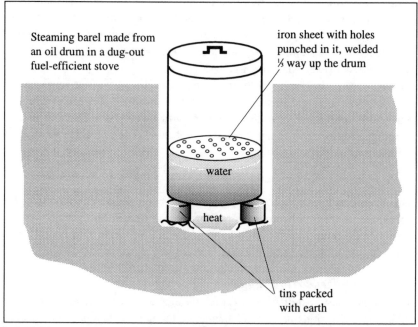

Steaming barel made from an oil drum in a dug-out fuel-efficient stove

iron sheet with holes punched in it, welded ⅓ way up the drum

water

heat

tins packed with earth

Insecticide treatment of clothes should be started if possible. People should be recruited to act as 'dusters' (employed to dust clothes with appropriate insecticide) to visit established households (1 duster per 150 households) and to work in the delousing centre for new arrivals (1 per 100 new arrivals per day). One supervisor will be required to inspect the work of every ten dusters.

Dusting gadgets can be made locally or bought commercially. A simple dusting 'sifter' can be made from a tin can by puncturing small holes in the base.

The implementation of louse and scabies control programmes are the only circumstances in which insecticide is deliberately applied to human bodies. It is important to use insecticides of the lowest suitable toxicity. If these are used then any minor side-effects experienced as a result of insecticide application are insignificant when compared with the levels of morbidity and mortality that may occur if treatment is not undertaken. The main considerations in choosing a suitable insecticide for louse control are:

• safety
• persistence

Implementing a control programme for lice

1 Inform the public that lice transmit serious diseases such as typhus and relapsing fever through their bite or via infective faeces, and elicit their support for the control programme. Inform people of the dangers of cracking lice between finger nails or teeth.

2 Change clothing every week especially underwear (away from human contact the lice will die). All members of a household should change their clothes on the same day, and clean clothes should be kept separate from dirty clothes. The NGO may need to provide clothing (especially underwear) to all or some of the population.

3 Heat dry clothing to 54^0 C for five minutes (all adults and eggs will die but care is needed to make sure that seams, waist bands, and pockets reach this temperature). This may be difficult to organise.

4 Boil or steam clothing for 15 minutes (wet heat is less effective than dry heat for killing lice but if left for 15 minutes most adults, larvae and eggs will die).

5 Treat clothing and bedding with insecticide. This can be done either by dipping clothing in an appropriate insecticide bath or dusting clothing. This will be effective against adults but not very effective against eggs, therefore treatment needs to be repeated after one week.

6 For a mass delousing campaign, administer 50gm of insecticidal dust (such as permethrin) to an individual through the neck band, waistband, sleeves, etc. of their clothing. Pay particular attention to seams and underwear where possible. For women either omit waistband treatment or employ women 'dusters' and ensure privacy. A 50gm measuring spoon or cup should be provided.

Care should be taken to delouse all feverish persons as well as corpses since lice from these persons will move on to a new host.

Head lice (P. humanus capitis)

Infection with head lice can cause considerable discomfort and, where infection is persistent, a malaise directly attributable to the infection can occur. Allergic reactions to lice faeces and saliva may also arise.

Control programme: Head lice infections can be controlled by using 'nit' combs, smearing the head with certain oils (e.g. coconut) and shaving. In many countries people shave the heads of children to control lice. Adults may also wish to shave their own heads for lice control. The provision of safety razor blades (1 per family) can be made where head lice infections are common.

Only pharmaceutical preparations of insecticide should be used for head lice control. People should be warned of the dangers of putting unsuitable insecticides in their hair (numerous deaths occur in developing countries as a result of the inappropriate application of agricultural insecticides to hair for head lice control).

Crab lice (Pthirus pubis)

Occurs on pubic hair and occasionally on beards and eyebrows. Fortunately crab lice are not associated with the transmission of any diseases.

Control programme: Shaving of pubic hair may be helpful. Only pharmaceutical preparations of insecticide should be used for crab lice control.

2.5 Tsetse-borne disease

2.5.1 Sleeping sickness (Trypanosomiasis)

Human sleeping sickness and animal trypanosomiasis (nagana) occur in Tropical Africa. They are transmitted by tsetse-flies (*Glossina* spp.).

2.5.2 Control programmes

Persistent organochlorine insecticides sprayed onto vegetation have been widely used to control tsetse. The spraying is restricted in height to the first 1.5m during the dry season and 3.5m in the wet season. Large numbers of refugees congested in one place are likely to have a major effect on the local vegetation, and this may reduce the tsetse population.

In recent years tsetse have been controlled using natural or artificial baits. Natural baits include cattle sprayed with insecticide. The tsetse population attracted to the cattle are killed, but not before they are able to bite the cattle and transmit nagana. Artificial baits include the use of traps and screens impregnated with insecticide that have been baited with an odour that is attractive to tsetse flies. The flies are killed either when they enter the trap or when they land on the surface of the insecticide-treated screen

Tsetse control is carried out in a number of African countries, (including Somalia, Uganda, Kenya, Zambia and Zimbabwe). Control is often directed at protecting cattle from nagana as this disease is of considerable economic importance. Outbreaks of human sleeping sickness are relative rare but when they do occur can be devastating. Control programmes will vary according to the particular tsetse vector which is responsible for transmission. Many

Table 8 Tsetse-flies as vectors of human and animal disease

Tsetse species	Disease	Control methods
riverine tsetse of West Africa	*Trypanosoma gambiense*	selective destruction of vegetation
	sleeping sickness in humans	insecticide spraying of riverine forests
		use of traps or insecticide treated targets
savannah tsetse of Sub-saharan Africa	*Trypanosoma rhodesiense*	selective destruction of vegetation
	sleeping sickness in humans nagana in cattle	insecticide spraying of savannah woodland
		use of traps and insecticide impregnated targets use of insecticide treated cattle

African countries have their own tsetse control department and these should be consulted whenever tsetse are thought to be a threat to the health of refugees or their cattle.

2.6 Bug-borne diseases

There are two families of bugs which are blood sucking: the bedbugs (*Cimex* spp.), and the cone-nosed bugs (Reduviid bugs).

Bedbugs
These bugs are renowned for their disturbing habit of biting at night, which may deprive people of their sleep. Bedbugs have also been implicated in the transmission of hepatitis B. They are often controlled as a side-effect of the use of insecticide-treated bednets for malaria control. The fact that bedbugs are also affected is a reason for the popularity of this method of malaria control.

2.6.1 Chagas disease

Chagas disease (American trypanosomiasis) is transmitted throughout the Americas and parts of the Caribbean by a reduviid bug via its infective faeces or via blood transfusions. The bugs are highly domestic and can build up large colonies in the walls, roof, and furniture of a house.

2.6.2 Control programmes

Control measures in the long term are based on improvements in housing (well-maintained brick walls and corrugated iron roofs) but where this is not possible, residual spraying will keep bug numbers down. Reduviid bugs are often controlled as a by-product of a malaria control programme.

2.7 Black-fly-borne disease

2.7.1 Onchocerciasis (river blindness)

This is caused by the parasitic worm *Onchocerca volvulus*. It is transmitted by blackflies (*Simulium* spp.) throughout much of Sub-Saharan Africa and is particularly severe in the savannah countries of West Africa. It is also found in small foci in Central and Southern America. The clinical manifestations of this disease include dermal, lymphatic, and systemic complications. The most severe complications include onchocercal lesions of the eye which may ultimately lead to blindness.

2.7.2 Control programmes

Until recently the only control method applicable at a community level was that of insecticidal control of the blackfly larvae which live in the 'white water' sections of fast flowing rivers. Repellents can be used to reduce biting nuisance. In most endemic countries in West Africa the Onchocerciasis Control Programme of WHO regularly treats the fast-flowing rivers that are favoured breeding sites of the vector.

The recent community-wide use of the anti-filarial drug 'Ivermectin' has proved extremely successful at reducing the symptoms of onchocerciasis but its effect on transmission is variable. The OCP (and its national collaborating partners if present) should be consulted if onchocerciasis is considered to be a potential threat to refugees in West Africa.

2.8 Sandfly-borne disease

2.8.1 Leishmaniasis

Leishmaniasis is a disease of humans and dogs infected with *Leishmania* parasites. There are three principal forms of the disease: cutaneous (e.g. *L. tropica*, usually self-healing); visceral (*L. donovani*, usually fatal if not treated); and mucocutaneous (*L. brasiliensis*, outcome variable). Different species of sandflies (*Phlebotomus* and *Lutzomyia* spp) are vectors of leishmaniasis, and also sandfly viral fever. The flies are associated primarily with rodents, dogs, and wild canines, but some species are peri-domestic and feed readily on humans. The inter-relationships of the various vectors, different forms of leishmaniasis, and animal reservoirs are very complex and often poorly understood.

In Southern Sudan the vector *Phlebotomus orientalis* is known to be associated with *Acacia-Balanites* woodland. Refugees have been infected with visceral leishmaniasis (kala azar) when passing through these woodlands at the end of the dry season. Refugee camps should not be sited within 1km of *Acacia-Balanites* woodland in an endemic area in Sudan and Ethiopia, and people should be warned about the danger of visiting such woods at dusk or night.

Since *P.orientalis* is known to bite in the early evening and at night, sandfly nets, especially when impregnated with insecticide, may be an effective measure for protecting individuals. These nets have a very small mesh size (sandflies are very small!) and are also effective against mosquitoes.

Termite mounds have long been associated with certain leishmaniasis vector species in east Africa (e.g. *P. martini* in Kenya) but their importance for *P. orientalis* is not clear.

2.8.2 Control programmes
Control measures against sandflies are effective where the flies are peri-domestic (in which case they are often controlled as a side-effect of malaria spraying campaigns) but are poorly developed for other situations. Some success has been achieved in reducing sandfly numbers in certain areas by destroying rodent colonies and thereby eliminating the flies' breeding and resting sites.

Table 9 Sandflies as vectors of disease

Diseases	Vectors	Animal hosts	Distribution
cutaneous leishmaniasis (severe dermal lesions)	*Phlebotomus* spp. (Old World) *Lutzomyia* spp. (New World)	disease reservoirs are rodents and other mammals	Widely distributed in Central Asia, the Indian subcontinent, Eastern Mediterranean, Middle East, Southern Africa and parts of Ethiopian Region, and Central and Southern America. Epidemics may occur where displaced populations are forced to live outdoors in proximity to rodent colonies or wild animals.
visceral leishmaniasis (kala azar) (fatal if not treated)	*Phlebotomus* spp. e.g. *P.orientalis* (Old World) *Lutzomyia* spp. (New World)	disease reservoirs are dogs, wild canines and humans	Occurs in Central Asia, India, South America, the Mediterranean basin, Sudan and East Africa. Epidemics are associated with war and famine.
sandfly fever (mild infection)	*Phlebotomus* spp. (Old World)		Mediterranean basin, Near and Middle East, Central Asia and South China.

Kala azar in Southern Sudan: 'Since 1984 an epidemic of visceral leishmaniasis (kala-azar) has been raging in the Western Upper Nile Province of Southern Sudan, and more recently in the east of the country, in Gedaref. The current epidemic is thought to have killed about 200,000 people in the last six years. Initially mistaken for an epidemic of typhoid, the disease was first correctly identified in 1988 by MSF-Holland, when doctors in refugee camps in Khartoum found numerous cases of the disease in persons displaced from the war zone near Bentiu.'

2.9 Mite-borne diseases

Mites are associated with disease either as vectors or, as in the case of scabies, as burrowers into human flesh. Both scabies and chiggers (mite larvae) infections can be extremely unpleasant because of the intense itchiness they cause. Secondary infections can occur as a result of scratching, and access to water and soap must play an important part of the control programme.

2.9.1 Scabies

Scabies is caused by the minute parasitic 'itch' mite (*Sarcoptes scabiei*) burrowing in the surface layer of a person's skin. Mites also cause 'mange' in a wide range of domestic and wild animals. The scabies mite is only active above 20^0 C, and is transmitted during host contact under warm conditions, for example, in bed. It is a major public health problem worldwide and can reach

Table 10 Mites as vectors of disease

Vector	Disease	Distribution
Sarcoptes scabiei	scabies	worldwide
Trombiculid mite	scrub typhus *Rickettsia tsutsugamushi*	restricted to Asia e.g. West Pakistan, Japan, tropical Queensland, Pacific islands
	nuisance bites by the larvae ('chiggers') cause intense itching	tropical and temperate regions of the world

epidemic proportions in refugee camps, where crowding and poor environmental conditions enable the mite which causes the infection to spread rapidly. It is related to shortage of water for washing and is *in theory* easily curable if instructions are carefully followed.

2.9.2 Treatment protocol for scabies

1 Sulphur ointment e.g. Tetmosal, Mitigal (10% adults, 2% children in yellow soft paraffin) is the method of choice as it is cheap, reliable, and safe to use on children and pregnant women. Three treatments are necessary.
2 Benzyl benzoate (25% aqueous emulsions is used) is effective but should not be used on infants, or males with scrotal eczema.
3 Benzene hexachloride (HCH) is effective with one application but contra-indicated for infants, small children, pregnant women, and in people with extensive lesions.
4 Permethrin has also been specially formulated for scabies control.

Treatment method
All treatments require that the entire body be covered with the emulsion, solution, or cream. No part of the body, from the chin downwards, should be left uncovered. In babies, the face, head, and neck must also be treated. When starting a treatment, start with the fingers, the spaces between the fingers, the hands, and the wrists, and rub in, or paint on, the emulsion or ointment thoroughly. Then do the same to the forearms, the upper arms, the armpits, axillary folds, shoulders, and back and front of the trunk. Women should play particular attention to the breasts and nipple area, and men and boys to the external genitalia. The buttocks, thighs, lower legs, soles of the feet, and toes should finally be treated. All these areas should be treated whether there are any spots to be seen or not, so that no part of the body is left untreated.

The treatment is best done at night before sleeping and, if possible, repeated the following night. Clothes and blankets should be changed the next day if possible. Allow 24 hours to elapse after the last treatment before bathing.

Everyone living in the same house should be treated at the same time, including people not related to the infected persons. Scabies control programmes must be carried out on a suitably large scale to reduce the likelihood of rapid re-infestation.

Reasons for failure of scabies treatment

1 Inadequate application of the chosen medicament: carelessly applied; applied only to obvious lesions; applied less often than recommended; washed off too soon; solution too dilute; other topical measures used simultaneously; incompletely used because of intolerance to the treatment.

2 Reinfestation: from untreated or incompletely treated household contacts or from unsuspected source.

2.9.2 Scrub typhus

Scrub typhus is a rickettsial disease transmitted by the larvae of trombiculid mites that parasitise rodents. Infections in humans can result in a high rate of mortality. The two main vectors (*Leptotrombidium akamushi* and *L. deliense*) have a wide geographical distribution within which they are patchily distributed in 'mite islands'. These islands are essentially 'man-made' and are those environments where field rodents have built up large populations, for example, in neglected areas of cultivation. In Malaysia, Sumatra, New Guinea, and tropical Queensland mite islands are associated with the coarse, fire-resistant grass *Imperata cylindrica* (kunai grass). Limited studies have shown that rat control may exacerbate scrub typhus transmission, because the mites, with fewer hosts upon which to feed, are more likely to feed on humans.

Scrub typhus: biological factors
* vector mites associated with rodents
* transmission occurs in mite islands
* control of rats may exacerbate human infection.

2.9.3 Control programmes

Destroying mite islands may be an effective control measure if the mites are first killed by spraying soil and vegetation with a residual pyrethroid insecticide spray.

2.10 Tick-borne diseases

Tick-borne diseases are fairly rare, and are unlikely to be a major hazard in a refugee setting unless as vectors of disease to refugee cattle.

2.10.1 Control programmes

Tick control of animals usually involves dipping the animal in an appropriate insecticide. Ticks are readily repelled by commercial repellents and may be controlled in houses during an insecticide campaign against malaria vectors.

Table 11 Ticks as vectors of disease

Vectors	Diseases	Distribution
softt tick (*Ornithodoros moubata*) whose lifestyle is similar to that of the bedbug	only important human disease is endemic relapsing fever (*Borrelia duttoni*)	throughout most of the tropics and subtropics, as well as North America and Southern Europe
hard ticks (*Ixodides* spp.)	tick paralysis resulting from toxins in tick saliva.	throughout the world but rare
	spirochaetal infections such as Lyme disease (*Borrelia burgdorferi*)	Europe and North America where it has recently caused an epidemic of arthritis
	rickettsial infections (such as Rocky Mountain Fever *R. rickettsia*).	North America
	viral infections such as Russian spring-summer encephalitis	widespread in Far East especially USSR

2.11 Flea-borne diseases

2.11.1 Murine typhus and plague

The two main flea-borne diseases, plague and murine typhus, are commonly transmitted between rats by fleas. These fleas may also bite other animals and humans and, in the process, transmit these diseases from the reservoir host. Over 220 different species of rat have been found to be infected with plague. In recent years murine typhus has been identified as the cause of fever in Khmers living at an evacuation site on the Thai-Kampuchean border.

The first signs of a plague outbreak may be an epidemic of the disease amongst the peri-domestic brown and black rats, with numerous deaths. This may be followed within two weeks by the first cases in humans. The explanation for the delay is that the vector transfers to the human host when a rat host is no longer available. This factor has very important connotations for plague control.

Plague: biological factors
- flea vectors associated with domestic rats
- epidemics most common in a humid environment at 10-29⁰C
- fleas don't survive when the saturation deficit is above 10.2 millibars
- control of vector *must* be undertaken *before* control of rats.

Jigger fleas (Tunga penetrans)
Imported from Latin America, this flea is now a serious pest in tropical Africa. The female jigger flea burrows into the soft skin of the foot and ankle in order to lay her eggs. The presence of a number of adult fleas in the foot can be crippling and often causes inflammation and secondary infections. If ignored these infections can lead to loss of toes, tetanus, and even gangrene.

Table 12 Flea-borne diseases

Vectors	Diseases	Distribution
the flea *Xenopsylla cheopis* associated with domestic rodents (the black rat *Rattus rattus* and the brown rat *R. norvegicus*)	murine typhus (*Rickettsia mooseri*); death rate can be significant (5%).	worldwide but most common in certain areas
fleas associated with rodents *X.cheopis* is a common vector in cities, ports and rural situations	plague (*Yersinia pestis*); the high death rate associated with this disease (up to 95%) is related to the poor nutritional status of the host	worldwide 35⁰S and 35⁰N.
X.brasiliensis is a common vector in rural situations		rural Africa, woody area of Bombay state
X.astia relatively poor vector found in villages, fields and ports		S.E Asia

2.11.2 Control programmes

Long-term control of fleas is best achieved by general sanitation measures and elimination of food sources, especially by rodent control. Flea control should always be considered when there is an active rodent control campaign since, when deprived of their normal host, fleas are likely to transfer to humans. Where a flea-borne disease is present or threatens, flea control *must* precede rodent control. Appropriate insecticidal dusts (such as permethrin or pyrimiphos-methyl) should be used in rat runs, burrows, and around dwellings.

Fleas may also be a serious nuisance-pest, causing considerable itchiness and consequently disturbing people when they sleep. Airing bedding may reduce flea numbers (fleas are very susceptible to desiccation) but insecticide control, using an appropriate insecticidal dust on bedding and furniture, is the only really effective method.

Control of jigger fleas is best achieved by wearing shoes but this option may be too expensive for refugees, particularly children. Once jiggers have become embedded in the skin they should be removed, as soon as possible, with a sterilised needle. If the extraction is done carelessly or in unhygienic conditions, secondary infections may result. Insecticidal dusts may be used to control jigger fleas but this is likely to be relatively expensive.

2.12 Rodents as disease vectors, reservoir hosts, and pests

The nuisance, health threat, and loss of foodstuffs resulting from rat infestations can be extremely serious in a refugee settlement. This is most often due to the unsanitary conditions that occur when large numbers of people are crowded together. An average rat (weight 100gm) eats 10 per cent of its body weight per day. If there is a large rat population the loss of food consumed and damaged by rats can be considerable. If the refugee settlement has been sited in an area where vector-borne disease is endemic in the wild rodent population, this disease can then spread to the refugees via the more domesticated rodents. The problems caused by rodents in refugee settlements can be summarised as follows:

- disease transmission
- consumption and spoiling of foods, clothes etc.
- destruction of nursery and vegetable gardens
- biting and disturbing people while they sleep.

2.12.1 Rodents associated with disease

Rats are associated with disease transmission to humans in a number of ways; for example, rat-bite fever is transmitted by a bite from a rat; leptospirosis is transmitted in rodent urine; and typhus and plague are transmitted from rats to humans by infected fleas.

Populations of wild rodents may invade human settlements when flooding has destroyed their burrows. Increasing contact between wild and domestic rodents is likely to increase the chances of disease transmission to humans.

Table 13 The role of rodents in disease transmission

Rodents	Mode of transmission	Disease
as vectors of disease	rat urine in water frequented by people (e.g. rice fields)	leptospirosis
	rat urine and saliva (often when food contaminated)	Lassa fever
	contamination of food or water by faeces of infected person or animal; rats may be very important source of infection	salmonellosis
	infection through consumption of infected rodents	toxoplasmosis
as disease reservoirs and hosts to parasite vectors	fleas	murine typhus plague
	mites	scrub typhus
	ticks or direct contact	tularaemia
	ticks	borrelioses e.g. endemic relapsing fever and Lyme disease
	ticks	rickettsioses e.g. Rocky Mountain Spotted Fever

55

2.12.2 Rodent proofing material

Mortar: 9 parts sand 1 part cement

Concrete: 4 parts coarse aggregate, 2 parts sand, and 1 part cement

Metal sheet: For attaching to woodwork such as the bottoms of doors and door frames, and for forming baffles on pipes, use galvanised sheet iron about 1mm thick.

Wire-mesh: For proofing ventilation points, use expanded metal or woven wire-cloth made from metal about 1mm thick, adequately rust-proofed and with a mesh size no larger that 6mm.

Paint bands: To prevent rodents climbing rough vertical surfaces, apply one coat of primer followed by two undercoats and finally one hard, high gloss coat. Very rough wall surfaces should first be rendered smooth with a mixture of sand and cement.

2.12.3 Control programme

Rodent control should primarily be based on camp-wide sanitation, including garbage disposal; trapping; and rodent proofing of food stores, stores for medical supplies, and buildings in general.

Providing rat-proof metal food boxes or rat-proof grain stores will help to reduce food loss. Rodent proofing of buildings can be achieved by the closing of all holes larger than 6mm (the smallest hole that a young mouse can enter) and stopping them with suitable rodent-proof material. Places to pay attention to are the gap under doors, holes where pipes or wire pass through walls, windows, and other openings used for ventilation.

Rat traps or snares are made throughout the world where rats are considered a nuisance (or are eaten). It is better to use a large number of traps over a short period in carefully chosen sites, than a few traps for a long period. Rats and mice can become 'trap shy'. An economic incentive can be introduced to encourage refugees to catch and kill rats (such as payment for rat tails). Particular attention should be paid to protecting vulnerable refugees (such as the old and sick) from being bitten by rats. Those suffering from leprosy may be especially defenceless when sleeping.

Rodenticides (oral poisons for rats and mice)

While rodenticides, if properly applied, may be a very effective way to get rid of rats or mice, their use in a refugee camp should be strictly limited — possibly to secure food stores. Only well-trained, experienced staff should use rodenticides. Many rodenticides are extremely toxic and if eaten can cause severe poisoning and even death. Because of the danger of such poisons, to children and animals in particular, this type of control is often totally unsuitable in a refugee camp.

People in refugee camps may use rats or mice to supplement their diet, and so it is important to be very sure that the animals are not being eaten in the camp before embarking on a rat-poisoning control programme. In some countries there are professional 'rat catchers', who feed their families on the rats they catch.

Cats and dogs will deter rats from entering a building but will have little effect on a population that has already built up.

Unless the environment in which the rats are living is also made unattractive for them, the rat population will return within a few months of the end of the control programme. Rat-roofing of buildings, and implementation of sanitation measures ,will not only be cheaper than a camp-wide rodenticide programme, but will also be a long-term solution if maintenance is kept up.

Rodenticides can be divided into two types: the acute poisons, and the anticoagulants, which will kill rats after one or more feeds (e.g. brodifacoum). Acute poisons (e.g. zinc phosphide), while restricted or banned in advanced economies, are often widely available in less-developed countries. Anticoagulant rodenticides (widely used in the USA and Europe) are much less toxic than the acute type, and accidental poisoning can be rectified by the administration of Vitamin K1 (but not K2 or K3).

If a rat-poisoning campaign is to be undertaken, then the anticoagulant type of poison should be used, and the control programme (which could last about three weeks) should be accompanied by a thorough and effective media campaign. The points to be made in such a campaign are:

1 Don't eat rats.
2 Deliver rat bodies to the collecting team.
3 Don't allow poison bait or dead rats to contaminate water or food supply.

Anticoagulants are administered to rats and mice using baits, such as cereals. These will normally have been dyed blue to indicate that they are not edible. Unfortunately, this may not be sufficient to deter people from eating poisoned grain (in parts of the Far East food is dyed blue for ceremonial and festive occasions). To discourage people from eating grain treated with rat poison use a rodenticide containing 'Bitrex', a very bitter, unpalatable compound which is added to many modern rodenticides. This makes the grain virtually impossible to eat and will greatly reduce the likelihood of accidental poisoning.

It is important that an environmental clean-up campaign should be conducted only *after* a trapping or poisoning campaign. You don't want to drive the rats away before they are exposed to poison, as they are then free to return.

The destruction of nearby wild rodent colonies, by gassing, or bulldozing their burrows, may reduce the likelihood of certain types of infection, such as cutaneous leishmaniasis; but remember, if the rodents are known (or just suspected) of being associated with flea-borne or mite-borne diseases, for example, murine typhus or scrub typhus, then the vector *must* be controlled *before* controlling the rodent. This can be done by dusting rodent burrows or rodent traps with insecticide.

Giant gerbils — a threat to Afghan returnees: 'Refugees returning to Afghanistan from Iran were housed temporarily in camps on the northern plains close to colonies of the giant gerbil — a major reservoir of cutaneous leishmaniasis. Had this not been in winter many hundreds of cases would surely have occurred.' (Ashford, LSTM personal communication)

3 Vector-control strategies

3.1 Introduction

The main factors to be considered in controlling vector-borne diseases in refugee settlements are as follows:
- choice of settlement site
- camp construction and organisation
- shelter
- community awareness and health education
- sanitation
- water-supply systems
- personal protection
- the use of insecticides.

These factors will now be considered in more detail.

3.2 Site choice

The decision as to where a refugee settlement should be placed is often made for political as well as practical reasons. If a choice of site is possible then careful consideration of possible sites in relation to disease vectors may be the single most effective way of controlling malaria, sleeping sickness, onchocerciasis, kala azar and tick-borne fevers. Guidelines for reducing vector-borne disease transmission by site choice and camp organisation are as follows:

1 Avoid areas of known vector foci (for example, breeding sites of malaria mosquitoes in marshy, swampy areas in Africa or the forest edge in Thailand; or of blackflies in turbulent rivers in sub-Saharan Africa).

2 Minimise likely vector-human contact (for example, by the provision of an adequate water supply away from the vector foci, and using screening material on doors and windows).

3 Minimise conditions which lead to increased vector populations (for example, by reducing potential breeding grounds such as poorly-maintained water supply systems, swampy ground, etc.).

4 Minimise conditions which lead to increased disease transmission (for example, overcrowding).

In some situations land may be available for refugees precisely because it has been abandoned by the local population on account of the prevalence of local disease vectors.

In South-East Asia it may be possible to reduce malaria transmission by *Anopheles dirus* by removing any forest growth within 2km of the camp. This land could be kept free of forest regrowth by using it for planting crops, or for such things as football fields.

An illustration of the effectiveness of site choice as an effective control measure: After 1980 many Khmers were denied refugee status in Thailand and were settled in camps on the Kampuchean side of the border, within the forested habitat of the jungle malaria vector Anopheles dirus. Camps were frequently evacuated as a result of fighting and relocated nearby; a process which had a major effect on malaria transmission in some camps. For example, the evacuation of Sok Sann camp to a new site within 6km of the previous camp resulted in dramatic reductions in malaria transmission and, according to Meek (1989) '...emphasises the potential for avoidance of malaria by appropriate siting of refugee camps when a choice of sites is available.'

3.3 Camp organisation

Since personal hygiene and community involvement in vector control are likely to be crucial factors in the control of vector-borne diseases, the factors which produce and encourage active refugee involvement in their own health care are also likely to have a major impact on the reduction of breeding sites for vector species (e.g. the construction and use of fly proof latrines or the removal of mosquito larvae breeding grounds).

In a comparison of refugee settlements run by the army, and those run with assistance from Oxfam and CIIR, in Nicaragua, Cuny (1977) found that, while there were no major health problems in the latter settlements (in which refugees were fully involved in camp planning and organisation) the army run camps were '...plagued with skin infections, various waterborne diseases and several outbreaks of minor contagious disease'.

The overall lay-out of a camp, the ease with which individual dwellings can be mapped, and the access routes throughout the camp, will all have an influence on the efficacy with which a control programme can be carried out.

3.4 Shelter

The availability of sufficient and effective shelter is of very high priority in setting up camps for refugees and displaced persons. Shelter is needed to protect people from the extremes of heat, cold, rain, and wind. Shelter in a refugee camp may vary from temporary flimsy structures which provide shade and little else, to traditional dwellings, houses, and tents. The materials used to construct shelters may be cotton fabric, mud, brick, concrete, wood, grass, palm fronds, or plastic. The type of shelter, where it is located, and the material of which it is built may affect vector-borne disease transmission in a number of ways:

1 Lack of sufficient shelter may result in crowding and the increased transmission of communicable diseases, such as typhus, which is transmitted by body lice.

2 Flimsy, open-walled structures may provide little protection from the entry of biting insects. Some vector species will not enter a solidly-built house.

3 Open-walled structures may not provide sufficient surface area for the spraying of a residual insecticide.

4 Cracks in masonry, and roofs of thatch may provide breeding and living habitats for certain disease vectors, such as reduviid bugs or bedbugs.

5 The siting of houses downwind and away from vector breeding sites may reduce the ease with which the vector can find its host.

6 The use of screens and curtains impregnated with insecticide will reduce the number of insects, especially mosquitoes, entering a dwelling.

7 A ceiling in a room can significantly reduce the number of mosquitoes by blocking their entrance from the eaves. The provision of material for ceilings can be considered as an important public health measure in some circumstances.

Insecticides vary in effectiveness depending on their formulation and the surface on to which they are sprayed. DDT and malathion, in wettable powder

(WP) formulations, have been widely used for malaria control by spraying as a residual deposit on to mud walls, thatch, and wood. Insecticides formulated to spray on fabrics are suitable for tent spraying.

Improving the quality of housing, either by providing corrugated roofs instead of thatch or by plastering walls, will reduce certain insect vectors and provide long-term control measures. Such improvements are expensive, and are often beyond the means of refugees themselves.

3.4.1 Termite damage to shelters

Termites can cause a considerable amount of damage to refugee camp buildings and dwellings where wood or plant material is used in construction. Repairs of termite damage can be expensive and time-consuming.

Termite-resistant timber

The most important method for termite control in buildings in the tropics is the use of termite-resistant timber. Such timber may be locally available and in many parts of the world is traditionally used in house building. A list of termite-resistant woods found in West Africa can be obtained from the Natural Resources Institute (see Appendix 1).

Preventing termite boring

To be effective, measures against termite boring *must* be initiated at the time of construction. Partial protection from termites can be achieved by treating the ends of the supporting posts that are placed in the ground, either by charring them, soaking them in sump oil, or painting them with creosote or copper-based wood preservatives. Another method is to bury wood ash in the post hole.

The most widespread method of termite control has involved the application of persistent residual organochlorine insecticides such as aldrin, dieldrin, and heptachlor. As a result of environmental considerations these chemicals are banned in many countries and are no longer so widely available; they are not recommended. Residual pyrethroids are effective termiticides when suitably formulated. All termiticides require very careful application, such as pre-treatment of timber and soil, and the possible hazards should be investigated. To treat a building after it has been constructed will not be very effective since the termites will be able to bore through those posts buried in the ground.

3.5 Community awareness and participation

The social cohesion, and political and structural organisation, of refugee and displaced communities vary according to the culture and recent political history of the community. Refugee communities may be rural peasants, nomads, or town and city dwellers, including the urban poor and the urban middle class. Those fleeing from civil war or political persecution may be highly politicised and socially structured, whereas rural farmers fleeing from famine-affected areas may have little social or political cohesion.

All vector control programmes require at least the passive if not the active participation of the refugees themselves. Wherever possible the refugee population should be the main source of labour in a vector-control programme and should be responsible for the development of and subsequent running of health promotion campaigns. Vector-control initiatives should, as with other health programmes, actively involve as many groups within the refugee community as possible, including teachers and schoolchildren, traditional leaders, religious groups, women's groups, military authorities, and community health workers.

Many different mediums can be used to get the message across, including radio, loud-speaker, songs, theatre, puppets, and billboards. Health messages should include information on the disease, its relevance to the refugee population, the control measures to be used, and how they will help to prevent the spread of the disease. Every attempt should be made to explain the need for the control programme and then to organise it in such a way that social and cultural requirements are met. *Remember: public support for a control programme is essential.*

UNHCR have developed an approach called 'people-oriented planning' which provides a framework for involving refugees in decision making. This approach is based on UNHCR's extensive experience, which shows that:

- Ignoring refugee resources (social as well as physical) undermines the ability of refugees to do things for themselves.
- It is usually more efficient in the short run, and always better for refugee capacity in the long run, to build on the patterns of work and distribution of resources that prevail in the refugee population.
- Work and programme patterns that are established in the first few days of an emergency are extremely difficult to change later on. For example, if women are not consulted by emergency staff at the programme's inception, then it may be impossible for planners to get the information they need to set up gender-sensitive programmes.

There are some circumstances in which health education is a particularly important aspect of a control campaign:

1 If the refugees are responsible for creating breeding sites. For example, the digging of shallow pits when collecting mud for house construction, in which water accumulates, can result in ideal mosquito breeding grounds. Discussions should be held with refugee authorities to decide on the most appropriate remedy. In some situations local legislation (either traditional law or local authority law) can be used against the creation of vector breeding sites.

2 If transmission of the disease is affected by cultural habits. For example, relapsing fever is most effectively transmitted when lice are crushed between the teeth or nails, enabling the spirochaetes to come into contact with the skin. Widespread public education on the dangers of such habits should be undertaken.

3 If the refugees themselves can effectively eliminate the breeding sites. *Aedes* mosquitoes, the vectors of dengue and dengue haemorrhagic fever, may be controlled by the covering of domestic water storage jars, and changing the water weekly. Again, widespread public mobilisation (possibly including legislation) is needed for effective results.

4 If the refugees effectively undermine insecticide campaigns. Residual insecticide spraying programmes for malaria control have faltered because householders have replastered or whitewashed newly-sprayed walls and covered up the insecticidal surface. Malathion, which is used for residual spraying, is often unpopular because of its smell. The mass control of body lice with insecticides requires that underclothing is thoroughly treated with insecticide. Women may be reluctant to be exposed to public delousing and the provision of private space may be important to the success of the programme.

5 If refugees can protect themselves from infection, for example, by using bednets or repellents.

3.6 Water supply

The availability of sufficient safe water for personal hygiene and domestic use is a very high priority in setting up a refugee camp. Water may be available to refugees either directly from rivers or swamps, via shallow or deep wells, or through a piped distribution system.

Collecting water may expose people to disease: When Chadian refugees were settled in the Poli Pehamba district of Cameroun it was feared that onchocerciasis, which was known to be endemic in the settlement area, could have a serious effect on a refugee population which had not previously been exposed to the disease. This fear prompted the call for assistance from an entomologist. He recommended that the refugee villages should be sited at a reasonable distance from the nearby river (where the vectors of onchocerciasis breed) and that water should be provided within the camp, in order to reduce the number of people visiting the riverside, where fly numbers were highest. (Walsh, 1981)

Refugees may store water in pots and jars for later use. The type of water supply system used and the condition it is kept in, may have a marked effect on the number of 'container breeding' mosquitoes. Control of mosquito breeding in overhead water tanks and cisterns can, in theory, be achieved using tight-fitting lids or small larvae-eating fish. Polystyrene beads (see later) have also been successfully used to control mosquito breeding in such situations.

The provision of piped water to community stand-pipes should reduce the need for household water storage pots, often the most important breeding site for *Aedes aegypti*. But if the use of water storage pots is the cultural norm then it may be difficult, without extensive discussion and education, to persuade people to change their habits. For this reason, most control programmes for *A. aegypti* rely on the use of insecticides; but there are only a few insecticides which may be safely used in drinking water.

3.6.1 Insecticides for treating drinking water

Insecticides approved by WHO for use in drinking water are:
* Temephos and pyrimiphos methyl: organophosphate insecticides of very low mammalian toxicity.
* Methoprene: a hormone that interferes with larval growth.
* *Bacillus thuringiensis* H-14: a bacterial insecticide.

No other insecticides should be used in drinking water.

Insecticides can all be formulated as slow-release briquettes, which gradually release the insecticide over a number of months. Alternatively they may be formulated with course sand granules, which also provide a slow-release system. The sand granules can be handled most easily if placed inside a fine nylon bag. Depending on the type of insecticide and the formulation these treatments should last between two and five months.

3.6.2 Water supply and mosquito control

Mosquito numbers can be controlled by careful water management. Measures include the following:

1 Remove mosquito breeding sites. Unblock gutters, empty water containers, including vases and animal dishes, on a weekly basis and scrub them out before refilling. Make sure that soakaways, septic tanks, and grease taps are tightly closed. Fill in any holes and cracks around their top. Drain or fill-in puddles where fresh water collects.

2 Prevent the excessive production of waste water. All piped water systems leak, and regular monitoring and repair of faulty pipes will reduce the production of stagnant pools. Water-saving taps can be used to reduce the wastage of water.

3 Find a use for waste water. Surplus water from stand pumps can be redirected into a vegetable garden. The amount of water required for washing is much greater than that required for drinking, and disposal of water after use may result in stagnant pools being created, or water being wasted in underground soak-away pits. Plants which are 'water hungry' such as eucalyptus, papaya, or banana, can be planted in the area of run-off, or by marshy ground, in order to absorb the surface water.

4 Screen or cover open water supply tanks to deny access to mosquitoes. Use rust-resistant material such as nylon, stainless steel or aluminium mesh.

5 Apply insecticides, that are safe for humans and animals, to drinking water. Slow-release briquettes of these insecticides are the most practical solution for use in water storage containers.

6 Larvivorous fish (i.e. fish that eat larvae) are used in some countries for controlling mosquito larvae in drinking water. This strategy is only feasible if there is already a programme in operation nearby.

3.7 Sanitation

Sanitation practices that are designed to reduce fly populations should take into consideration the fact that flies breed in all kinds of decaying organic matter (human and animal food waste, excreta, corpses, and rotting plant material). The choice of sanitation system will depend on a number of factors, such as the speed of provision, the number of people, and the resources available, the traditional defaecation practices, and the height of the water table.

The high rates of malnutrition and mortality related to diarrhoea in infants and younger children of Kurdish refugees (12 per cent of all children died within the first two months of the crisis) took place rapidly despite prompt relief efforts and a previously healthy population. This experience emphasises the need for early and aggressive public health management of sanitation, water sources, and diarrhoea control programmes to augment the traditional focus on food and medical relief during the emergency phase of a refugee crisis. (Yip and Sharp, 1993)

The type of sanitation system used may have a marked effect on fly numbers and also on the types of fly that will breed. Unless particular measures are taken to prevent fly breeding then the introduction of a sanitation system may actually *increase* fly numbers by providing permanent, damp, warm environments that are suitable habitats for flies to breed in.

There are several ways of preventing flies breeding in organic matter:

1 Incinerate rubbish, hospital dressings, and dried manure. In some situations animal manure may traditionally be used as a fuel source. If the dung is thinly spread and dried quickly, then fly numbers should not be excessive.

2 Prevent flies getting access to potential breeding sites. This may be achieved by burying garbage and faeces in a trench and covering it with a minimum of 25cm of compacted soil.

3 Localise the organic matter in such a way that flies breeding in it are unable to escape. For example, the ventilated pit latrine is designed to prevent flies escaping.

4 Treat organic matter with an insecticide. Filth flies are notoriously susceptible to developing insecticide resistance so this method should only be used *if absolutely necessary* and then only for a short time.

A well-organised, highly motivated, well-supervised defaecation system will ensure that defaecation is restricted to the proper sites and that latrines are kept clean and well-covered.

3.7.1 Types of defaecation system

Different defaecation systems will affect both the number and type of flies that occur.

Indiscriminate defaecation throughout the camp: some filth flies, including *Musca sorbens*, which is commonly found feeding on eye secretions, are adapted to breed in small piles of human faeces. Over 42,000 larvae have been found in 1kg of human faeces. Covering faeces with a thin layer of soil may actually *increase* the fly population, because the breeding habitat will remain moist. Flies are attracted to faeces by smell and, if necessary, will burrow down into loose earth to lay their eggs.

Defaecation fields: these should be chosen to be at least 500m up wind from any habitation or feeding centre and at least 30m from the water supply. Defaecation fields will produce as large a number of flies as would indiscriminate defaecation but, if fields are sited up wind, the numbers of flies flying into the camp will be reduced. Washing facilities should be available nearby. Defaecation fields will localise excreta, making it easier to clear up. A large workforce will have to be employed to clear the fields and dispose of the excreta in prepared pits; it should then be covered with 25cm of compacted soil. The workers will require protective clothing.

Wind location may change frequently or seasonally. In Africa the wind usually changes direction at the beginning and end of the rains, and therefore defaecation fields should either be changed in accordance with wind changes or the site should be chosen to be up wind during the period of maximum fly numbers. Ask local inhabitants when flies are most common.

Dry latrines: trench latrines, and any other ordinary latrine where faeces are piled together, provide an ideal breeding site for filth flies such as blue-bottles and green-bottles and less so the important *Musca* spp.

Trench latrines should be filled daily with compacted soil to a depth of at least 25cm to prevent flies breeding.

Fly proofing of latrines

Tightly-fitting lids: fly breeding can be reduced by making sure that well- fitting lids are used to cover the latrine hole. Wooden or sheet metal lids are likely to warp and therefore become ineffective. Sacking soaked in motor oil and used to cover the latrine hole will provide some protection from fly breeding.

Pour flush latrines: the water seal prevents the escape of smells from the latrine and also prevents the entry or departure of any insects. Such latrines are only appropriate where people use water, and nothing else, for anal cleansing. As for the ventilated improved pit latrine, this type of latrine must be perfectly sealed to be effective.

Ventilated improved pit (VIP) latrine: the VIP latrine is characterised by the presence of a ventilation pipe which draws odours away from the pit thus reducing unpleasant smells. If the latrine is fitted with a roof and is fairly dark inside, then flies breeding in the pit will try and leave the pit via the vent pipe and can be trapped in it by a wire mesh at the top. Flies will try to enter the latrine via the vent pipe — where the smell is strongest — but will be

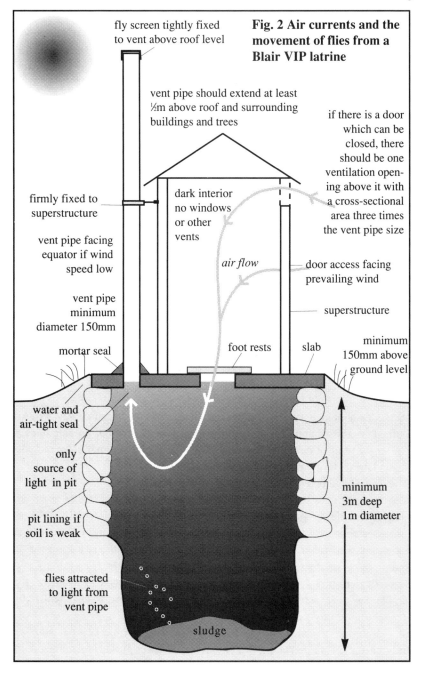

fly screen tightly fixed to vent above roof level

Fig. 2 Air currents and the movement of flies from a Blair VIP latrine

vent pipe should extend at least ½m above roof and surrounding buildings and trees

if there is a door which can be closed, there should be one ventilation opening above it with a cross-sectional area three times the vent pipe size

firmly fixed to superstructure

dark interior no windows or other vents

vent pipe facing equator if wind speed low

air flow

door access facing prevailing wind

vent pipe minimum diameter 150mm

superstructure

mortar seal

foot rests

slab

minimum 150mm above ground level

water and air-tight seal

only source of light in pit

pit lining if soil is weak

minimum 3m deep 1m diameter

flies attracted to light from vent pipe

sludge

prevented from doing so by the wire mesh. The main disadvantage of the VIP latrine is the cost of the vent pipe, which may be 90 per cent of the total cost of the latrine. In the Thai-Cambodian border camps VIP latrines were made using large bamboo pipes, painted black inside.

Latrines must be carefully constructed and well-maintained if they are to be effective at controlling flies. The main factors for ensuring the effectiveness of a VIP latrine are:

- the vent pipe must be of the correct size (150-200 mm) and work efficiently
- the pipe must be fitted with a corrosion resistant screen (e.g. stainless steel or aluminium)
- semi-darkness is essential within the covering structure
- the latrine hole should not be covered
- the latrine should be kept clean
- there must be no cracks in the masonry.

While in theory VIP latrines are simple to build and should provide effective fly control, in fact, they are often poorly constructed, badly sealed, and do not live up to their reputation.

VIP and pour flush latrines, if carefully constructed, will also provide effective control of the urban nuisance mosquito, *Culex quinquefasciatus,* the vector of bancroftian filariasis (elephantiasis). Malaria vectors will only breed in unpolluted water and will therefore not be found breeding in latrines.

Reducing mosquito breeding in wet latrines
Insecticides should *never* be used inside the latrine pit because they will kill benefical organisms and thus prevent the natural breakdown of organic matter.

In a new refugee camp, mosquito control should be automatically included in *every* latrine during construction when:

- the water table is reached during latrine construction
- seasonal rains are very heavy and likely to cause water to lie in latrines
- large quantities of sullage water will be poured down the latrine.

In an established camp all latrines should be inspected and only the 'wet' ones ear-marked for treatment. There are three main methods to prevent the breeding of mosquitoes:

Use of dry material: the weekly addition of dry material to a latrine (for example, sawdust, ash, lime, or powdered earth) may absorb sufficient liquid to prevent mosquito breeding.

Oil: old engine oil can be poured into the pit latrine (one cup per standard family latrine). This makes the water surface of a wet pit latrine an unsuitable place for mosquito larvae to breed in as they are unable to breathe. This can be an expensive use of oil, may not be effective on heavily polluted water, and must be repeated weekly to be effective. Oil should not be poured into latrines if there is the possibility that it may contaminate water supplies. Waste from latrines where engine oil has been used should be carefully disposed of and should not be composted for agricultural use. (A series of technical notes on the construction of pit latrines and their vent pipes is produced by the Intermediate Technology Group.)

Polystyrene beads: polystyrene beads (just like those found in bean bags) have been used in vector control programmes in east Africa to prevent mosquitoes from breeding in wet latrines. The beads can be purchased in their unexpanded form, in which they are easier to transport. When they are heated to 100°C in water over a fire they swell to 15–20 times their original size (this process does not use CFCs). Steam treatment results in even greater expansion. The expanded beads are then poured into the latrine. They form a surface cover over the liquid which allows faeces to fall through but makes it impossible for mosquitoes in the water to emerge. If the water dries out, then the beads settle but they are rapidly refloated should the latrine fill with water again. These beads can also be used in water storage tanks.

Although, in theory, a layer of polystyrene beads should last indefinitely, they may be lost from the latrine during flooding or pit clearance. The risk of the beads being lost, and the possible environmental consequences, should be considered before implementing the use of beads as part of a control programme.

The use of expanded polystyrene beads for mosquito control in wet latrines: A 2cm layer of 2mm beads is sufficient to eliminate mosquito breeding. Thus, 20 litres of expanded beads are needed per square meter of water surface, or 30 litres for a typical pit latrine. This weighs about 1.25kg if expanded in boiling water and costs about $2.50. Expansion in boiling water uses about 0.05m³ of firewood to produce 240 litres of expanded beads. This takes two to three hours from lighting the fire. Using this system it is estimated that 1.5 tonnes of polystyrene beads will be sufficient to treat 2000 latrines. (From Curtis, et al., 1991)

3.7.2 Screening

Screening of buildings is an important way of preventing disease transmission by flies and mosquitoes. Rust-proof (stainless steel or aluminium) mesh should be used in hospitals, feeding centres, and especially kitchens. If mesh is not available then 'fly doors' (made of strips of plastic or fibre) will help to reduce fly numbers.

3.7.3 Garbage collection

Garbage containers must be available throughout the camp and especially in the market area. Garbage should be collected daily if possible, but at least every three days, to reduce fly breeding. Collected garbage should then be burnt or buried in a deep pit or landfill site and covered with a minimum of 25cm of compacted soil. The more compact the garbage the fewer flies it will produce. If garbage is not disposed of, this will encourage rat populations to build up.

Garbage containers should be metal, and perforated at the base and supported off the ground to allow rain water to drain. 200 litre oil drums that are sawn in half are ideal for this task. If no containers are available, plastic sacks may be used as a temporary measure.

3.8 Environmental sanitation

3.8.1 Water

Water engineers employed to organise the water supply in a refugee settlement should also have a responsibility for reducing mosquito breeding sites through 'environmental sanitation'. This includes the drainage of swampy areas, land levelling, the removal or planting of vegetation in or near swampy areas, and the building of dykes. Such control methods can be very effective and long-term solutions. Much of the small-scale, physical work can be carried out by the refugees themselves. A number of texts on vector control that are suitable for engineers are listed in the references at the end of the book.

3.8.2 Vegetation

Removal of vegetation within and around the borders of the camp may be useful for the control of 'mite islands', if these can be identified, and provided the vegetation is not mostly of crops. The destruction of a band of woodland around a settlement in a tsetse-infested area may reduce the threat of human and animal trypanosomiasis since tsetse-flies are reluctant to fly over open spaces. This control method has been used extensively in Africa and is known to be reasonably effective. In Africa there is a widespread belief that malaria vectors commonly breed in the leaf axils of maize plants: this is *not* the case.

3.9 Personal protection

There are a number of ways in which individuals can protect themselves from vector-borne diseases. They include:
* personal hygiene and behaviour
* suitable clothing
* use of bednets
* use of repellents.

These will now be looked at in more detail.

3.9.1 Personal hygiene, behaviour, and clothing

Regular washing of body and clothes, the use of soap, protecting food and cooking utensils from flies, and careful use of latrines will reduce considerably an individual's exposure to fly-borne pathogens and lice, as well as reducing the chances of secondary infection of insect bites. Individuals can reduce their own exposure to mosquito, blackfly, sandfly, tsetse, and tick bites by wearing long clothing (such as trousers and long sleeved shirt or long dress) or clothing impregnated with insect repellents (see section 3.9.4). Personal cleanliness can be enhanced by the provision of soap, or soap-making facilities, to the refugee population.

3.9.2 Bednets

Bednets (mosquito nets) are used widely throughout the world (especially in the Far East) depending on mosquito nuisance, tradition, availability, and affordability. Other motives for using bednets are: privacy, and protection from cold, rats, gheckos, cockroaches, or spirits. In very hot climates bednets may be uncomfortable to sleep under because they reduce ventilation.

Bednets and malaria

Bednets are widely used because they reduce the nuisance of mosquito bites. Since many malaria vectors bite people at night, when they are sleeping, bednets can also reduce people's exposure to malaria. A recent study in The Gambia showed that malaria prevalence levels were *inversely related* to mosquito vector density. The researchers concluded that this was because people in areas where there were a lot of mosquitoes protected themselves with bednets. However, in areas where malaria transmission is more intense, ordinary bednets may not reduce mosquito biting enough to affect malaria transmission.

The effectiveness of the use of bednets for malaria control, as with any other control method, will be dependent on public support and co-operation. If the refugees are not familiar with the use of bednets then a carefully organised experimental trial should be initiated first, to assess their acceptability and effectiveness.

Provision of bednets

The questions to ask when considering bednets for vector control are:
* Are mosquitoes considered a major biting nuisance?
* Are the disease-carrying vectors normally biting people while they sleep?
* Are bednets widely used by the local population? If not why not?
* Are bednets normally widely used by the refugee population? If not why not?

Poor quality nets deteriorate quickly and do not stop mosquitoes biting. NGOs may play an important role in the provision of effective bednets (either free or at cost price) in a refugee situation, as well as encouraging their use by the host population. Providing suitable netting material to local tailors (or refugee tailors) will provide employment as well as a supply of bednets; but local tailors may not be able to produce large numbers of nets quickly in an emergency.

Bednets can be bought locally, in which case they are likely to of a type familiar to people, but care should be taken to buy nets of a good quality otherwise their effectiveness will deteriorate rapidly. Cotton nets are usually the most comfortable but they are liable to rot in humid conditions and are more expensive than nylon, polyester or polythene nets. Polyethylene nets are the strongest type and, with proper care, should last up to five years. Nets made from 40-denier polyester are widely used in Asia but are very flimsy and are not recommended for refugee situations. The greater effectiveness of the more expensive, higher-denier nets (75-100) with borders is well worth the extra cost. Bednets may be a fire hazard and people should be warned not to smoke in bed when nets are used.

Cot, single, and family bednets can be bought as well as large communal nets. The size of net chosen should be in accordance with sleeping habits and space available. Many imported nets come from Thailand or the Philippines, where they are widely used. A family-size net should cost less than $5.00 (including shipping costs). Bednets may vary considerably in quality and style between manufacturers, so be sure to investigate your sources thoroughly before placing an order. A list of major manufacturers is given in Appendix 2.

Bednets are unlikely to provide complete protection from malaria for the following reasons:

- mosquitoes bite people before they go to bed, when they get up in the night, or when they rise in the morning
- mosquitoes can get inside nets that are not properly tucked in or are torn
- mosquitoes bite parts of the body which lean against the net
- hungry mosquitoes unable to feed from one person may feed instead on their unprotected neighbour.

Insecticide-treated bednets

This idea is not new. Egyptian fishermen in the fifth century BC were known to keep off mosquitoes while they slept by covering themselves with their oily nets (the fish oil presumably acting as a repellent). A surge in popularity of bednets treated with insecticide (usually pyrethroid) is currently under way. Widespread trials throughout the world (in particular China, Vietnam, Solomon Islands, Papua New Guinea, Burkina Faso, Tanzania, Kenya, and The Gambia) have shown it to be a useful technique that is practical in community-based projects and is effective against both nuisance biting and malaria transmission. Insecticide-treated bednets have been shown to reduce child mortality substantially in The Gambia, but their effectiveness in areas of higher malaria transmission is not yet clear.

Insecticides used for net impregnation

Photostable pyrethroids are chosen because of their low toxicity, rapid insecticidal effect, and long residual efficacy. Permethrin-treated bed nets have been endorsed by the WHO Expert Committee for Malaria and are least likely to cause any problems of skin irritation during dipping. Deltamethrin, lambdacyhalothrin, and other more recently developed pyrethroids are effective at lower concentrations but may cause temporary skin and nasal irritation.

Choice of insecticide should depend on availability, safety, persistence under environmental conditions, and cost. Good quality formulations which are specifically for bednets should be used. Agricultural permethrin should *not* be used as it will have been prepared using different solvents, which may reduce the safety and acceptability of the treatment. Individual treatment sachets for nets (which expatriates can use to treat their net before travel) can be obtained from the Schools of Tropical Medicine in London and Liverpool. Pre-impregnated bednets can now be purchased in a number of camping shops. They will be of particular benefit in an emergency situation but the means to re-impregnate them must still be organised in the field.

Washing bednets

Washing the treated bednet will reduce the amount of insecticide on it (sometimes to nil) so it is recommended that bednets should be laundered before re-impregnation with insecticide, every six months. This problem needs to be clearly understood by the refugee community. Wash-proof formulations of insecticide may be on the market soon.

Bednets and other vectors and pests

Sandflies: mosquito nets are not usually fine enough to prevent the entry of sandflies, which are extremely small insects. Where sandflies are a major biting nuisance, 'sandfly nets' may be found which are made of opaque sheeting. The effectiveness of these nets can also be improved by treating them with a residual pyrethroid insecticide. A mosquito net that has been treated with insecticide will kill or at least repel sandflies trying to enter it.

Bed bugs and head and body lice: immediately after insecticide impregnation the bednet should be left to dry on the sleeping mat or bed of the owner. The residual effect of any pyrethroid that is left on the bed should eliminate bedbugs for up to two months and also reduce the prevalence of head and body lice.

Protocol for insecticide-impregnated bednet programme

Materials required:
  pyrethroid E.C,
  plastic bucket(s)
  protective gloves
  inert measuring cup
  insecticide syphon

To calculate the strength of the permethrin emulsion needed:

1 Calculate absorption of netting:

  The amount of water absorbed by a net will depend on the type of cloth. For an average nylon family size net this may be 500ml whereas, for a cotton net, this may be 1.5-2 litres. It is therefore important to calculate the average amount of water used to soak an individual net if you want to dip nets *en masse,* or to work out the amount of water absorbed per net if they are dipped one at a time.

  Let is assume the average amount of water absorbed is 500ml

2 Calculate amount of pyrethroid a.i. needed per net to give recommended dose cover/m

The surface are of the net is:

(w x h x 2) + (l x h x 2) + (w x l x 1) + (area of overlap if any) = xm

w = width, h = height; l = length.

For an average single net this may be 10m²

Treatment of 100 nets of 10m² area requires:
1 litre of permethrin 50 per cent E.C. in 249 litres water @ 0.5gms a.i./m
1 litre of deltamethrin 2.5 per cent in 249 litres water @ 0.025g a.i./m
400ml of lamdacyhalothrin 2.5 per cent in 249.6 litres water @ 0.001g a.i./m

After dipping, the nets should be gently squeezed to remove excess liquid and then laid out on a flat surface (preferably the mattress) to dry. If the nets are dried outdoors they must be spread out in the shade as sunlight will break down the insecticide. When dry, the net is ready for use. Nets should normally be impregnated immediately before the main malaria transmission season. If transmission occurs throughout the year then re-impregnation should usually be undertaken every six months.

Cost
Estimated cost is less than $0.50 per treatment. Treatment will be required 6-12 monthly depending on the pyrethroid chosen and control circumstances.

A preparation to treat a single net is available from some manufacturers and may be particularly suitable for NGO staff to use before leaving to work in a refugee camp.

3.9.3 Insecticide-impregnated curtains
The use of insecticide-treated curtains for malaria and leishmaniasis control has been tried experimentally in a number of situations. Curtains are particularly suitable for use where people do not normally use bednets and are unlikely to adapt them to their current way of living. Unlike impregnated bednet programmes, there is as yet little information as to the efficacy of the use of impregnated curtains as a control measure. Before embarking on an impregnated-curtain programme a carefully controlled experimental trial would be required.

3.9.4 Repellents

Insecticide-treated bednets and repellents are essential to safe-guarding the health of aid workers exposed to certain disease vectors.

Traditional repellents

Throughout the world people use a variety of different substances to reduce the annoyance of insect biting. They use methods such as burning dung, citrus peel, or other material in the evening when mosquitoes are biting, or rubbing oils (such as turmeric or mustard oil), ash, or plant juices on the skin. Common traditional treatments for headlice include rubbing neem or coconut oil on to the scalp. Such well-known practices should be encouraged, for example, by the provision of a simple oil-extraction press. Some traditional repellents are known to be very effective, although there are many which have not been evaluated scientifically. It should be noted that not all natural products are completely harmless and, where possible, further information on possible side-effects should be obtained.

Mosquito coils

These remain smouldering for four to six hours but may be too expensive for many refugees. The quality of mosquito coils varies considerably, and there are many on the market that are not effective at all. Pyrethroid-based coils are more effective than those using natural pyrethrins alone.

Commercial repellents

Deet (Diethyltoluamide) is the best known commercial insect-repellent and is widely used in commercial products. It will repel mosquitoes, sandflies, blackflies, chiggers, ticks, deer flies, and fleas. The concentrated Deet should be diluted to 25 per cent in a suitable solvent (e.g ethanol, isopropanol, petroleum jelly, or solvent-based cream) and smeared on to the exposed skin surface. It should act as an effective repellent for six hours. Applied to the skin it offers hours of protection but when absorbed onto clothing it usually provides protection for several days. It is relatively cheap if bought in large quantities ($9.00/kg). Other effective commercial repellents are Dimethyl phthalate and Dibutyl phthalate.

Permethrin repellent bar

This soaplike bar (which costs about $0.30/bar direct from the manufacturers) is an effective repellent if used correctly. The user should rub the bar on their exposed skin in the evening and not wash it off until the morning or until ready to go under a bednet to sleep. One bar may last up to a month if carefully used.

Choice of repellent

Trials by Lindsay (1989) in The Gambia on the use of different repellents against blood-seeking mosquitoes showed that soap with deet (with or without permethrin), burning santango (traditional Gambian repellent), or a mosquito coil all provided reasonable degrees of protection The choice between these treatments is primarily a question of convenience and cost.

3.10 Insecticide control programme

There are three basic methods of using insecticides for control of insect vectors and pests. The choice of which technique to use depends on the target insect, the life stage to be controlled, and the various technical advantages or disadvantages of each technique.

3.10.1 Residual spraying

Residual spraying of a suitable insecticide is the recommended technique for malaria control where the vector is known to rest indoors. Table 14 gives details of spraying programmes which might be appropriate. Residual spray programmes are relatively simple to organise but must be well-supervised. The roles and responsibilities of a spray team are given in Table 15. Spray teams should spray all the dwellings, and sometimes the animal sheds as well, once or twice a year (see Table 2, p.26 for operational indicators used in malaria control). (Using a residual insecticide on bednets is not included here as it has already been covered earlier on.)

Table 14 Residual spraying of insecticide

Residual spray	Target insects	Notes
this consists of applying a suitable insecticide to a surface upon which the vector/pest is known to rest long enough to pick up a lethal dose	indoor resting mosquito vectors and indoor feeding sandflies	indoors – the standard recommended technique for indoor resting mosquito vectors
	Triatomine (cone-nosed) bugs	indoors – the standard recommended technique for triatomine bugs
indoor treatments are usually done with a hand-held compression sprayer while outdoor treatments are usually done with power-operated sprayers	household pests (bedbugs, cockroaches, fleas, ticks)	indoors
	flies	not recommended for fly control as likely to increase development of resistance
	tsetse-flies and sandflies body lice, bed bugs, fleas	outdoors – needs to be applied to vector resting sites (trees, termite hills) applied as a dust

Table 15 Members of residual spray team for malaria control

Personnel in residual spray team for malaria control	No.per team	Tasks
Supervisor	1	supervise the field team, undertake simple health education
Spraypersons	4	spray the insecticide
Mixer	1	collect water, mix the insecticide prior to adding it to the spray tank (not needed where pre-packed sachets of insecticide used)
Insecticide distributer		collect, weigh and package insecticide

3.10.2 Larviciding

Larviciding programmes can be technically simple to do, and can be easily organised provided there is sufficient supervision.

Larvicides may be applied by hand-carried, vehicle-mounted or aerial equipment. Applications may need to be repeated at intervals of 7-14 days depending on circumstances and the type of larvicide used. Table 16 gives details of appropriate methodology. Fuel oil can be used as an effective larvicide, but will be expensive as relatively large amounts of oil are required (150-200litres/ha) when compared with larvicidal oils (20-50litres/ha).

Table 16 Larviciding

Larviciding	Target	Notes
should only be applied when and where breeding has been shown to occur; the operator/supervisor must be able to recognise the target insect	'container breeder' mosquitoes (e.g. *Aedes*)	the recommended method for mosquitoes breeding in artificial containers which cannot be controlled in another manner (see section 3.6 for mosquito control in drinking water)
should only be adopted where vector breeding cannot be limited by environmental or sanitation measures (such as draining, filling, destroying or covering breeding sites)	other mosquitoes	an important control technique where the extent of mosquito breeding is within the economic control capabilities of the control programme
	blackflies	the only vector-control technique against vector blackfly species but must usually be done over a large area otherwise the breeding site will soon be reinvaded by migrant blackflies

3.10.3 Space spraying

Thermal fogging with 2-5 per cent malathion or a synthetic pyrethroid will give effective control of adult mosquitoes if the fog can penetrate to where they are resting. Pyrethroid insecticides have the advantage of tending to irritate insects and encouraging them to fly. Thermal fogs are usually applied by ground equipment such as the hand-held or shoulder-carried pulse-jet machine or a two-stroke engine-exhaust fog generator. Vehicle-mounted fogging machines are also available.

Aerial space spraying is usually done with the ULV (ultra low volume) method using the same insecticides (but as different formulations; see section) as used in fogging programmes. Ground spraying with ULV can be achieved by modifying the normal fogging machines by restricting the flow of insecticide and removing the heating section.

Space spraying must be restricted to an hour or two in the early morning or evening, when the temperature is lowest and thermal currents, which cause excessive dispersion of the insecticide, are at a minimum. If done at other times, the programme will be considerably less effective.

4 Insecticides

4.1 Introduction

To the inexperienced, the list of chemicals that can be used to control a particular insect pest or vector can seem bewildering. The important factors to be considered when purchasing insecticide are:
- suitability
- registration in country of use
- availability
- safety
- degree of resistance developed to the insecticide by the target vector
- compatibility with spray machinery
- cost (including transport, application system, and protective measures).

4.2 Suitability

Deciding on a suitable insecticide will depend on a number of factors. For an insecticide to be useful it must affect the target organism to such a degree that the transmission of the disease is considerably reduced. This requires familiarity with the properties of a particular insecticide (the active ingredient) and the ecology and behaviour of the target insect (including general habits of the species, the particular life-stage, and previous insecticide history). This information is summarised in Table 17.

Information about the correct formulations, dosages, and application techniques should be obtained from the manufacturers of the different insecticides. The types of insecticide to be used for particular control programmes, and their usual dosage per area, can be found in a number of WHO publications.

Table 17 Common insecticides[1] for use against important public health vectors

Insecticide	Vector groups				
	Mosquitoes	Houseflies	Lice	Fleas	Bugs
Organochlorine DDT[2]	✔	✗	✔	✔	✗
Organophosphate Malathion	✔	✔	✔	✔	✔
Fenitrothion	✔	✗	✗	✗	✗
Temephos	✔	✗	✔	✗	✗
Pirimiphos methyl	✔	✗	✔	✔	✗
Carbamate Propoxur	✔	✗	✔	✔	✗
Pyrethroids (Natural) Pyrethrin	✔	✔	✗	✗	✗
Pyrethroids (Synthetic) Bioresmethrin	✔	✔	✗	✗	✗
Permethrin	✔	✔	✔	✔	✔
Cypermethrin	✔	✔	✔	✔	✔
Deltamethrin	✔	✔	✗	✔	✔
Lamdacyhalothrin	✔	✔	✗	✔	✔
Tetramethrin	✔	✔	✔	✗	✗

1There are other suitable insecticides available on the market – careful consideration should be given to choosing the most suitable for the task.
2DDT is banned in many countries because of the its effect on the environment. It is, however, still widely used in public health programmes in some countries because of its low cost and relatively low human toxicity.

Table 18 Common insecticide formulations used in vector control

Formulation	Notes
Wettable powder (WP) (water soluble)	Most common formulation for residual spray for malaria control. Usually contain 50 per cent or more active ingredient. Should not be mixed with an emulsifiable concentrate. Widely used where there is a range of substrate type (mud, thatch, brick, concrete). Where the substrate is porous or is coated with organic material, a wettable powder formulation should be used.
Water dispersible granules or grains (WDG)	These products which are beginning to replace the old-style WP, may be conveniently formulated as tablets or unit pack sachets which can be placed directly into the sprayer's tank. They therefore reduce the level of exposure of the handler/mixer to the insecticide.
Emulsifiable concentrate (EC) (emulsion suspension in organic solvent)	Usually contains 2.5-25 per cent active ingredient. Should not be used in ULV as solvent is too volatile. Used for residual spraying on painted walls (where people object to white deposit left by WP).
Suspension concentrates (SC)	These are aqueous suspensions of a particulate insecticide or (if microencapsulated) of liquid insecticide droplets. They have the advantage over ECs in that organic solvents (which can be inflammable or toxic) are not used.
Fog formulations (may be thermal or cold fog)	Uses an oil-based insecticide solution (which may pose a fire hazard). Pesticides which have a fumigant action are ideal. Great care must be used to avoid inhaling fogs. Operators should use respirators.
ULV (ultra low volume)	Best option for fast control in an epidemic but since ULV formulations are often very concentrated, care must be taken to ensure safety of operators and public.
Dust	Storage problems often occur in humid climates.
Granules	Used in larviciding as they do not drift as much as space sprays. Suitably formulated with sand they can act as slow-release formulations.

4.2.1 Quality control

Insecticides may be of poor quality because they were either poorly manufactured or incorrectly stored, or they were adulterated. There are some simple precautions that can be taken to ensure that the insecticide is of good quality:

• only buy from well-known manufacturer
• always buy new stock
• buy insecticides manufactured to WHO specifications
• have the insecticide tested by an independent analyst
• transport and store according to manufacturer's specification
• protect from theft and adulteration.

4.2.2 WHO specifications

The quality of an insecticide for use in public health programmes can best be ensured by using only insecticides which have given satisfactory results in all four phases of the WHO Pesticide Evaluation Scheme (WHOPES) and which comply with WHO specifications. Since many vector control programmes take place in remote areas, these insecticide formulations may have to be stored for considerable periods under tropical conditions and during this time they must remain in a satisfactory state for immediate use. The active ingredients must not deteriorate and the physical properties, particularly the suspensibility, must not become impaired. For example, the malathion wettable powder specifications (WHO/SIF.10.R5) includes a heat-stability treatment designed to exclude powders that could form an impurity hazardous to sprayers and other workers. Details of WHO insecticide specifications can be found in *Specifications for pesticides used in public health,* WHO (1985) and subsequent issues for specific products and formulations.

Independent analyst

The quality of an insecticide can be verified on purchase by sending a sample to an independent analyst. If needs be standardised reference insecticide samples can be obtained from WHO for use by local analytical laboratories.

4.3 Registration

The great majority of the world's pesticide usage is against agricultural pests. There are far fewer insecticides suitable for use in public health programmes. These are limited to chemicals which have been found to be of sufficiently low mammalian toxicity to permit their safe use on or near human beings. The relatively small public health market means that insecticide companies do not necessarily register their products for public health use, even when they have been shown to be safe and effective for the control of a particular disease vector. It is these complex commercial interests, combined with differences in national registration policy in both exporting and importing countries throughout the world, that produce the confusing situation where certain insecticides are available in one country but not in a neighbouring country. Some countries have highly sophisticated registration procedures which every insecticide formulation must pass before it can be used; whereas other countries are still in the process of developing their registration procedures.

Registration of a particular formulation of insecticide by a company will nearly always be specific to a trademark, a container, a formulation, and in some cases other features, such as the country of manufacture.

To find out which insecticides are registered for what purpose contact the local Registrar of Pesticides, or staff within the Ministry of Health, such as the Malaria Division, or the Public Health or Sanitation Department, or (often the most useful) the Department of Agriculture. The local agents of insecticide companies within the country should also be able to provide information on products, and their assistance in following registration procedures, clearing customs, and organising transport should be sought.

Unregistered insecticides
Insecticides may not be registered because:
* they are considered inappropriate or dangerous for a particular problem;
* there has not been sufficient commercial interest to warrant registration.

4.4 Availability

Insecticides may not be available in certain countries because of registration restrictions. Large quantities of insecticide from major manufacturers may take several weeks to supply. If they then have to be transported to the country of use, further delays will take place in transit (if the insecticides are not registered then the delay may be permanent!). Planning in advance is essential.

If insecticides are to be purchased locally then be sure that they are from a well-known supplier and that they are not out-of-date stock. Do not use insecticides which are not labelled with a description of the active ingredients. The brand name alone does not provide enough information, because different chemicals are sometimes sold under the same brand name.

Preparedness: Rodent and flea control in the Thai-border camps was initiated to control murine typhus but, more importantly to test whether the control measures would be sufficient if ever plague was introduced into the camp. Meek (1989) explained the problem:
'...Although plague has not been reported in Thailand for over 40 years it has been found recently in Burma and Vietnam and would require swift action in a crowded camp with dense populations of rats and fleas. It was found that most insecticide dusts were not registered for sale in Thailand as there was no market for them, and dusting equipment had to be specially made. Such setbacks emphasize the need for clearly prepared plans for control of diseases which have not yet been reported.'

The Pesticide Index
This is an essential reference source, annually updated, which tells you at a glance the active ingredient, brand name, and marketing company of almost any pesticide you might encounter. Also included is an address list of companies around the world who market pesticides. It is published by the Royal Society of Chemistry.

(Non-profit making organisations, such as NGOs and educational establishments, in countries eligible for UK aid, can obtain a copy of the *Index* free of charge from the Natural Resources Institute.)

4.5 Insecticide safety

Some insecticides are much safer to humans and the environment than are others.

4.5.1 Toxicity
The toxicity of an insecticide is given as the dose required to kill 50 per cent of a sample of test animals in a specific time, and is referred to as the Lethal Dose 50 (LD50). Thus *the lower the LD50 the greater the toxicity of the insecticide.*

This form of classification is of limited value, as insecticides will vary in their toxicity to humans and animals according to various factors, such as the percentage of active ingredient in the formulation.

4.5.2 Level of hazard

The same insecticide poses different hazards to mammals depending on how it is formulated and whether it has been ingested orally or absorbed through the skin. In general, solid formulations (dusts, wettable powders) are less hazardous than liquid formulations of equivalent toxicity.

WHO have developed a classification of different insecticides on this basis, as shown in Table 19. Preference should be given to the least hazardous insecticide suitable for the control purpose. The hazard classification is a better guide than the simple LD50 quoted in many textbooks but is as yet not widely used.

Table 19 WHO insecticide classification of acute hazard

Class level Acute Hazard		Oral toxicity		Dermal toxicity		User restriction category*
		Solid	Liquid	Solid	Liquid	
1a	Extremely Hazardous	<5#	<20	<10	<40	1
1b	Highly Hazardous	5-50	20-200	10-100	40-400	2
11	Moderately Hazardous	50-500	200-2000	100-1000	400-4000	3
111	Slightly Hazardous	>500	>2000	>1000	>4000	4
U+	Acute Hazard unlikely					5

mg/kg body weight
+ Unclassified
* Based on LD50 for the female rat (mg/kg body weight).

User restriction categories are:

1 Only individually licensed operators.

2 Specifically trained, educated and strictly supervised operators.

3 Trained and supervised operators known to observe strictly prescribed precautionary measures.

4 Trained operators who observe routine precautionary measures.

5 General public respecting standard hygienic measures and observing labels.

4.5.3 Guidelines on pesticide safety

Safe handling of pesticides involves trying always and everywhere to minimise the risk of exposing oneself and the environment to the undesirable effects of these poisons.

Safety instructions for handling pesticides
* read the label and follow instructions carefully
* wear clean and appropriate protective clothing
* never leave pesticides unattended in an insecure place
* never transfer pesticides to inappropriate containers, especially beverage bottles
* inspect pesticide containers for leaks and handle them with care
* do not keep food, drink, tobacco or eating utensils in the work area
* never eat, drink, rub your eyes, or touch your mouth while working with pesticides
* always have soap, water and a change of clothing available
* always discard heavily contaminated clothing and faulty protective covering, especially gloves and respirators
* if leaks or spills occur, decontaminate immediately
* keep unauthorised persons (especially children) away from pesticides.

The safety of refugee adults and children should be considered during all phases of an insecticide-based control programme. Where residual insecticides are being used, all householders should leave the room, taking all food items with them, before spraying begins; and water containers should be securely covered. Householders should only be allowed to re-enter the room once spraying has been completed.

Useful literature on pesticides
Literature on all insecticide products used by an organisation should be kept at headquarters as well as in the field. A number of useful publications are available for general guidance.

Wherever possible local guidelines (based on internationally accepted guidelines) that cover specific control programmes should be produced in the local language.

GIFAP is the International Group of National Associations of Manufacturers of Agrochemical Products. It produces a number of booklets and posters related to the safe use of pesticides including *Guidelines for the safe and effective use of pesticides*; *Guidelines for the safe transport of pesticides*; and *Guidelines for personal protection when using pesticides in hot climates*. These guidelines are straightforward simple texts for field use, and are highly recommended. They can be obtained from GIFAP (address Appendix 1).

4.5.4 Safe transport of insecticides

Insecticides should not be transported in lorries carrying food. If this is unavoidable small quantities can be placed in a separate compartment (such as a lockable metal or wooden box). Care should be taken to protect containers from damage or theft. Drivers should be instructed to keep insecticides separate from food, safe from children and animals, and secure from theft. Drivers should be instructed on emergency procedures in case of an accident. These are:

* switch off engine and disconnect battery
* do not smoke
* avoid skin contact or inhalation of fumes
* contain small spills by covering with earth or sand
* if there is a large spill of concentrated insecticide then remain by vehicle (upwind) and send for assistance
* prevent insecticide from contaminating water system
* keep public away.

4.5.5 Safe storage of insecticides

Insecticides should *always* be stored separately from food stuffs, and under lock and key. A secure insecticide store should be constructed wherever insecticides are used. The insecticides must be protected from heat, cold, and damp if they are to remain in good condition. Organophosphate insecticides such as malathion can convert to more toxic chemicals if they are stored at high temperatures.

4.5.6 Safe disposal of insecticide containers

In all tropical countries, and in refugee camps in particular, the empty pesticide container is valuable for other uses. Large metal containers have been flattened to provide building materials and drums have been used to collect and carry water. People have died as a result, because pesticide containers can never be made sufficiently clean to be safely used for food or drink.

All containers should be washed out several times and the rinsing added to the spray. The containers should be punctured before being buried in a deep pit (at least 1.5 m in depth) preferably in clay soil, and well away from a water source. If the insecticide is diluted in organic solvents, the container should be washed out with kerosene before being buried.

4.5.7 Safe disposal of unwanted insecticide

Few countries in the tropics have incinerators which are capable of destroying insecticides safely. The need to destroy insecticides usually arises for one of three reasons:

- the supply of inappropriate insecticides
- the oversupply of insecticides
- the deregistration of insecticides.

Insecticides are sometimes deregistered (i.e. permission for their use withdrawn) as countries tighten their environmental protection regulations. The insecticides most likely to be deregistered are the persistent organochlorines such as dieldrin, heptachlor, and DDT. Extreme care should be taken when disposing of unwanted insecticide. The advice of the manufacturer should be sought as to the safest method of disposal.

4.5.8 Protective clothing

Protective clothing is required *whenever* insecticides are handled. The type of clothing needed for different levels of operation is described in Table 20. When the safest insecticides are used, a change of clothing, and ample supplies of soap and water for washing may be all that is required; but gloves, goggles, respirators, and aprons may also be needed. In tropical countries some types of protective clothing may be too uncomfortable to use and will increase the amount people sweat, which in turn increases their ability to take up pesticides through the skin.

Protective clothing can be a major source of exposure to operators if it is not either carefully washed or disposed of after use. The least toxic insecticides should always be considered first.

4.6 Treatment of pesticide poisoning

4.6.1 Exposure to pesticides

Exposure to pesticides can be limited in the workplace by the provision of protective clothing, water, and soap, and training vector control staff in the safe handling if pesticides.

Monitoring exposure to organophosphates

If a long-term pesticide programme is being set up, all persons exposed to, or involved in, the handling, processing or spraying of an organophosphate compound should be checked weekly for a depression in the levels of

Table 20 Types of protective clothing that may be required

Protective clothing	Mixing concentrate	Residual spraying	Fogging
apron disposable leather, PVC	required with all Class 11 or above. recommended for Class 111		
fire blankets			where oil based solvents used
footwear impermeable shoes or boots (i.e. not canvas)	minimum requirement	minimum requirement	minimum requirement
clothing head to foot clothing including long trousers and long sleeves; change of clothing	minimum requirement	minimum requirement	minimum requirement
ear protection ear plugs, earmuffs cap-type ear muffs			must be worn with larger fogging/ULV machines
face shields	essential where dusts or liquids used	when spraying	when spraying
gloves solvex, PVC nitrile, neoprene	minimum requirement but **only** if carefully washed or discarded	minimum requirement **only** if care- fully washed or discarded	minimum requirement but **only** if carefully washed or discarded after use
goggles (anti-fog)			when spraying
hats (with large rim or peak)		when spraying	when spraying
respirators (with carbon filter) dust mask, hoods respirators			suitable for use when fogging; filters need changing regularly
safety spectacles	when certain solvents used		when certain solvents used

cholinesterase (an enzyme found in the blood that is deactivated by organophosphorus compounds). A pre-exposure cholinesterase level must be determined for all personnel before they come in contact with the insecticide. This will serve as a base line for assessing any decline in the level during spraying operations. Anyone showing a drop of 50 per cent or more from the base line pre-exposure level should be removed from contact with the insecticide until the cholinesterase returns to the baseline levels. Test kits for measuring cholinesterase are available commercially.

4.6.2 Operational staff

All those involved in an insecticide or rodenticide operation should be aware of the symptoms of accidental poisoning and the immediate treatment protocol. Information on these must be included in any training programme. Posters and written guidelines must be made available in the local language. Staff should be able to demonstrate that they know exactly what to do in an emergency.

Safety instructions for dealing with pesticide poisoning
All staff should be fully aware of the following simple rules to follow in case of pesticide poisoning:
- Remove patient from contact.
- Act calmly, keep patient comfortable and strictly at rest.
- Remove contaminated clothing, wash exposed skin thoroughly.
- Pay attention to breathing, give artificial respiration if required.
- Lay patient on his or her side.
- If highly toxic material has been swallowed, induce vomiting (only in conscious patients).
- Get medical assistance.

4.6.3 Information for medical staff

Guidelines for treatment of pesticide poisoning should be available in the appropriate language in the central health centre of any refugee camp along with the antidotes required. Staff should be aware of which insecticides or rodenticides are being used in the area (for vector or pest control) and the action that needs to be taken in cases of poisoning. GIFAP produce a set of guidelines: *Guidelines for emergency measures in cases of pesticide poisoning* (GIFAP 1984).

Antidotes
Antidotes (where available) to any pesticides used in the camp or surrounding area should be held in the medical centre. These include:

- activated charcoal for use if pesticides have been swallowed
- atropine sulphate, for exposure to organophosphates (ESSENTIAL)
- pralidoxime chloride, for exposure to organophosphates within 12 hours of poisoning
- diazepam, to reduce anxiety
- phenobarbitone, to reduce anxiety
- Vitamin K1, for use with anticoagulant rodenticides.

4.7 Insecticide resistance

A number of different factors can contribute to the failure of a vector control programme and one such factor is resistance of the insect to the insecticide. Other factors are usually more common and they need to be investigated first should control failure become apparent. The factors which may be involved in the failure of mosquito control programme are:

- inadequate operation methods
- poor quality spray application
- low rate of insecticide coverage
- mosquito behaviour (e.g. remaining outdoors)
- insecticide resistance.

Insecticide resistance to certain insecticides is widespread in mosquitoes, lice, and filth flies. Before purchasing an insecticide for use against a particular insect in a particular part of the world, check with national or international sources on the likelihood of insecticide resistance occurring. Companies will not accept liability for the failure of a control programme if it is due to insecticide resistance. In all insecticide programmes, the susceptibility of the insects to the chemical used should be tested regularly (i.e. annually). WHO store and make available information on all cases of proven resistance reported to them, and produce a useful publication on this subject

4.7.1 WHO susceptibility test
The standardised susceptibility tests developed by WHO should be used to test for insecticide resistance. This technique uses standardised insecticide-impregnated papers placed in an exposure chamber. The target insects are introduced into the tube and exposed to the insecticide for one hour. They are then removed and placed in a second chamber and their recovery over a 24-hour period is observed. The same system has been adapted for a number of insects and impregnated papers for testing are available for a number of

different insecticides at a range of doses. While the technique itself is simple to understand, its practical application in a field situation depends on the user having a good understanding of the scientific problems associated with it.

Several factors are likely to influence the apparent potency of an insecticide, such as the sex and age of the insect, and environmental conditions, especially temperature, and thereby affect the results of a resistance test, and so standardisation of the test is very important. Insecticide susceptibility tests that are not correctly carried out may give misleading results and seriously affect the efficacy of the control programme.

4.8 Cost of insecticide

Most companies have complex pricing structures and there may be little flexibility in insecticide purchase price for voluntary agencies. It may be easier to negotiate about the services attached to the insecticide order (such as provision of machinery, consultants, and back-up services). When calculating the cost of a particular insecticide or spray machine it is important to take in to account all the other factors affecting costs: personnel, frequency of spray round, protective clothing, shipping, etc. The book *Guidelines for cost effectiveness analysis of vector control*, Phillips, M, Mills, A, and Dye, C (1993) is again recommended.

4.8.1 Donations of insecticide

Offers of donations of insecticide should be treated with caution. Only accept those insecticides that would normally be considered acceptable and are appropriate for the particular problem to be tackled. Donated insecticides should be analysed to be sure that they meet the requirements of safety and efficacy.

Companies may donate insecticide or spray equipment in order to tie an organisation into their 'system', by being obliged to buy spares or replacements from them. The full implications of accepting donations should always be carefully considered.

5 Selection of spraying equipment

5.1 Choosing the right equipment

Having made a decision to put into operation a vector-control programme which involves the spraying of insecticide, it is important to make sure that reliable and appropriate equipment is obtained. The factors governing the selection of spraying equipment fall into three categories:

1 Operational factors
- target insect
- speed required to treat area
- area requiring treatment
- availability of labour
- characteristics of area
- frequency of application.

2 Factors related to machinery
- complying with WHO specifications
- compatibility with available machinery
- durability
- ease of use
- availability of spare parts
- availability of after sales service
- availability of diluent.

3 Cost factors
- transportation
- operating costs
- capital investment required.

These factors will now be considered in more detail.

5.2 Operational factors

In an emergency the most immediate control strategy against adult mosquito vectors (i.e. during a dengue, yellow fever epidemic) or filth flies is by rapid application of insecticide in the form of a space spray (aerosol) through which the insects fly.

Space spraying can be organised and undertaken much faster than a residual spraying programme, and can be administered from the air under certain circumstances.

Space spraying will also be effective against adult mosquitoes much faster than a larviciding programme which will not eliminate the adult mosquito population for up to 30 days. The type of machines to be used for space spraying will depend on the size of the area which requires coverage. (This may be considerably diminished if careful examination of epidemic information suggests that transmission is fairly focal.) Larger, more powerful machines can cover a much greater area very quickly but this must be balanced against other factors.

Table 21 Estimates of average daily coverage of different space spray delivery systems

Twin-engine aircraft/large helicopter	6000 ha
Light fixed-wing aircraft/small helicopter	2000 ha
Vehicle-mounted cold-fog generator	225 ha
Vehicle-mounted thermal fogger	150 ha
Back-pack mist blower	30 ha
Hand carried thermal fogger	5 ha

(Taken from Brès, P (1986) *Public Health Action in Emergencies caused by Epidemics.*)

5.2.1 Size of machinery
When deciding what size of machine to purchase there are certain operational constraints which will affect the decision:

1 Availability of vehicle and fuel for vehicle-mounted machine
  a. in an emergency
  b. during the normal transmission season.
Remember that tractors and other vehicles may have many other urgent uses.
2 Accessibility of camp to vehicle-mounted sprayer. Is the terrain suitable?
Are the tents or houses far enough apart to allow access? If the vehicle cannot
move readily throughout the various sections of the camp, then many places
will not be sprayed. The spray cover on either side of the vehicle will vary
depending on wind speed and direction.
3 Availability of labour
  a. in an emergency
  b. during the main transmission season.
Remember that to do the same job, several small machines will require many
more personnel to operate them than one or two larger ones.

5.3 Factors related to machinery

5.3.1 Availability of machinery

Before any purchases are made it is essential to first find out what is available
within the host country in the way of suitable spray machinery, spare parts, and
after-sales service. Importing machinery is expensive, and there may be long
delays in the supply system and in customs, so *early planning* is essential to
ensure that the machinery will be available when needed. If machinery can be
purchased locally, make sure that the supplier is reliable, that spare parts are
available, and that the machine is of a suitable quality.

A detailed guide to types of machinery can be found in *Equipment for
Vector Control*, WHO (1993). This book also gives details of the WHO
specifications for different types of machinery, such as WHO/VDC/89.970:
specifications for hand-operated compression sprayers; and
WHO/VBC/89.973: specifications for thermal fogging equipment. By using
these specifications as a guide, the purchase of unsuitable machines can be
avoided.

A list of machines and their manufacturers which comply with WHO
specifications can be obtained from CTD/WHO.

The International Pesticide Application Research Centre (IPARC), has the
largest collection of spray machinery in the world and can be contacted for
advice on different types of machinery. The book *Pesticide Application*

Methods, by Matthews (1992) is an essential general reference text on pesticide spraying techniques and indispensable for the technical person in charge of spray programmes (especially those involved in fogging).

The most commonly used spray equipment for vector control is the hand-operated compression sprayer, especially for indoor residual spraying. These sprayers are simple to use and have also been widely used for applying larvicides and molluscicides for schistosomiasis control. Those that comply with the WHO specifications have been used extensively in malaria control programmes around the world and, if carefully maintained, have a satisfactory field life of up to ten years, even when heavily used. One of the problems associated with a compression sprayer is that, as the insecticide is discharged, the pressure in the tank changes, resulting in an uneven rate of application. This can be avoided by using a pressure regulator but these often become clogged with insecticide.

Spray Management Valve

A new development in this area is a Spray Management Valve (SMV), which is an automatic pressure-regulating valve that is designed to fit every type of knapsack or compression sprayer on the market. It will greatly improve accuracy in spray delivery, and should reduce wastage and accidental exposure of operators to spray. (It costs around £10 and is highly recommended.)

5.3.2 Compatibility

Some machines are designed to be compatible with nozzles and spare parts of other manufacturers. Compatibility will save both time and money when spare parts are needed.

5.3.3 Diluent

Different machines are designed to use different diluents for the insecticide a.i. In many cases the diluent is water, and a supply of clean water must be made available to the spray team because dirty water will block the filter and damage the nozzle. In the case of thermal fogging, diesel or kerosene is used as the diluent, and these must be made available to the spray programme and their cost included in the overall control programme costs. In areas where water is in short supply ULV (ultra low volume) sprays should be used if possible.

5.3.4 Maintenance

Equipment will degenerate rapidly unless properly maintained.

Ease of maintenance is an important criterion in selecting equipment.

Preference should be given to equipment on which components subject to wear are readily accessible for easy replacement. Since some insecticide formulations may corrode or otherwise damage the spray equipment, manufacturers should be consulted about the compatibility of the insecticide formulation with the materials used in the construction of the application equipment. Equipment and machinery for insecticide application should be stored in a secure, dry area. Rubber components should be protected from rats.

Copies of manufacturers' guides to the spray machinery and the machine motor should be available in the field and in the head office to facilitate ordering of spare parts. Unfortunately, many manufacturers seem unaware of the conditions under which their equipment may be used in the field, and manuals, where available, seldom give enough detail to be useful in practice. They are rarely translated into languages other than that of the country of manufacture.

Guides to general maintenance of spray machinery should also be obtained for use in the field. The tools necessary for routine maintenance should be sent to the field with the machines. Regular maintenance will ensure that the sprayers are in working order when needed and will save money by reducing the need for spare parts and new machines.

5.3.5 Availability of spares

Preference should be given to equipment for which basic spare parts are readily available. Some basic spare parts (for example, nozzle tips, washers, 'O' ring seals and other replaceable components) should be bought at the same time as the equipment to avoid delays in spraying during the control programme. Poor quality spare parts (especially those made of rubber) may wear out in a couple of days' field operation. Brass nozzles wear out quickly when WP formulations are used.

Reliability is a factor in choice of machinery: if 50 per cent of 20 small machines break down then spraying can still go ahead. if a single large machine breaks down then no spraying at all can be undertaken.

Do not buy machines of poor quality

The use of WHO recommended spray equipment will prevent purchases of poor quality machines. Macdonald (Entomologist UNBRO) describes how poor quality machines are used as scrap to make dusters to dust rat burrows for flea control '...The dusters are made from the pumps of old spray cans that did not work out in the DDT program. (While expensive, we use Hudson X-pert and have a warehouse full of other, broken, brands of sprayers).'

5.4 Cost of machinery

The cost of machinery must be included in the overall cost of a control programme. The easiest to maintain, most robust machine that is compatible with the level of servicing available, the size of the area to be controlled, the speed necessary for control and the availability of labour will be the machine of choice. There is considerably price variation between apparently similar machines.

Beware of false economy: cheap, poor quality machines may prove more costly in the end in terms of insecticide wastage, the need for frequent servicing and replacement of parts, and possibly even the failure of the control programme. Good quality machinery will only remain so if basic maintenance is regularly undertaken. The addresses of some major firms involved in the supply of application machinery are given in Appendix 2.

The table opposite gives details of the recommended control method, and the appropriate equipment, for the most common disease vectors and pests:

Table 22 Guide to equipment suitable for application of insecticides for some vector control operations

Vector	Recommended control method	Equipment used for control
MOSQUITOES *Anopheles* spp.	interior residual treatment	hand compression sprayer, stirrup pumps
	interior space spraying	intermittent or continuous hand-operated aerosol dispensers, portable aerosol generators or mist blowers, mosquito coil
	exterior space spraying	power-operated mistblowers, aerosol generators, aircraft ULV equipment
	larviciding	hand- or power-operated granule applicators, hand compression sprayers, knapsack sprayers, aircraft spray and granule equipment
	bednets	impregnated netting
Aedes aegypti and *Aedes albopictus*	space spraying	ground-operated small aerosol disperser, portable power aerosol generators or mistblowers
	larviciding as for *Anopheles* spp except that dusters and granule applicators are seldom used	
Aedes simpsoni	exterior space spraying	power-operated mistblowers, aerosol generators, aircraft ULV equipment
other *Aedes* and *Psorophora* spp.	as for *Anopheles* spp. except that interior residual spraying is not used	
Culex spp.	as for *Anopheles* spp. except that interior residual spraying is of limited use	

103

Vector	Recommended control method	Equipment used for control
Mansonia spp	interior residual treatment	hand compression sprayers, stirrup pumps
	vegetation control	hand- or power-operated sprayers for herbicide application
SYNANTHROPIC FLIES		
Musca spp. *Stomoxys* spp. *Chrysomya* spp. and *Calliphora* spp	interior (cattle sheds and pig sties) and exterior (waste dumps) residual treatment	hand compression sprayers, power-operated sprayers, stirrup pumps
Lucilia spp.	interior space spraying	intermittent or continuous hand sprayers, aerosol dispersers or generators
	interior trap	sticky baits
	exterior space spraying	power-operated mistblowers, aerosol generators, thermal foggers
	larviciding	hand- or power-operated sprayers
Glossina spp.	exterior residual treatment	hand-operated compression or knapsack sprayers, power-operated vehicle mounted sprayers
	exterior space spraying	power-operated mistblowers, aerosol generators, aircraft spear or ULV equipment
	traps, screens	monoconical or biconical impregnated traps, screens
Simulium damnosum complex	larviciding	aircraft spray equipment
Other *Simulium* spp.	exterior residual spraying	ground aerosol generators, power-operated mistblowers, aircraft spray equipment

Phlebotomus spp *Lutzomyia* spp.	interior residual treatment	stirrup pumps, hand compression sprayers
	exterior residual treatment	power-operated vehicle mounted sprayers
Culicoides and *Leptoconops* spp.	interior residual treatment	stirrup pumps, hand compression sprayers
	exterior space spraying	aerosol generators, power-operated
	larviciding	hand- or power-operated sprayers and granule applicators, aircraft spray and granule equipment
Chrysops and other tabanids	exterior space spraying	aerosol generators, power-operated mistblowers, aircraft spear and ULV equipment
	larviciding	hand- or power-operated sprayers, aircraft spray equipment
FLEAS *Xenopsylla* spp and *Pulex* spp.	interior residual treatment	hand-operated dusters and sprayers
Ctenocephalides spp.	interior and exterior residual treatment	hand-operated dusters and sprayers
BEDBUG *Cimex* spp.	interior residual treatment	hand-operated compression sprayers
REDUVIID BUGS Domestic spp.	interior residual treatment	hand-operated compression sprayers
LICE *Pediculus humanus capitis*	hair treatment	hand-shaker, dusters and shampoo

Vector	Recommended control method	Equipment used for control
Pediculus humanus corporis and *Phthirus pubis*	clothing and body treatment	Hand-operated dusters and sprayers
COCKROACHES	interior residual treatment	hand-operated dusters and sprayers
TICKS and MITES Ixodids	interior residual treatment	hand-operated dusters and sprayers
Argasids	interior residual treatment	hand-operated sprayers and dusters
Trombiculids	exterior residual treatment	hand- and power-operated dusters and sprayers, power-operated mistblowers, aerosol generators, aircraft spray equipment

Taken from WHO (1990) *Equipment for Vector Control*

Appendix 1
Addresses of relevant organisations

Centre for Disease Control and Prevention (CDC)
Public Health Practice Program Office
Atlanta GA 30333
USA
Fax: (1) 404 488 7772
This centre has expertise in the biology and control of a range of disease vectors.
Request information on training materials from:

Distance Learning Program CDC/Public Health Foundation
P.O. Box 753 Waldorf MD 20604
USA
Fax: (1) 301 843 0159

Centre for Research on the Epidemiology of Disasters (CRED)
Catholic University of Louvaine
Ecole de Sante Publique
Clos Chapelle-aux champs 30
Brussels B-1200
Belgium
Tel: (32) 2 764 3327
Fax: (32) 2 764 5322
Telex:B 23722 UCL WOL
This centre works mainly on the impact of disasters on health. CRED have self teaching slide sets on disasters and public health.

Central Science Laboratory,
Formulations Analysis Section,
Ministry of Agriculture and Food,
Hatching Green,
Harpenden,
Hertfordshire AL5 2BD.
UK.
Fax: (44) 582 762 178
Telex: 826363
This institute can provide a list of analytical laboratories in Europe.

Famine Early Warning System
USAID FEWS Project
Tulane Pragma Group
1611 N Kent St. Suite 1002
Arlington VA 22209
USA
Tel: (1) 703 522 722
It is possible to obtain some higher spatial resolution Landsat images for certain parts of the world through the Famine Early Warning System (FEWS). Where these images are available they can often be obtained for the cost of reproduction from:

Earth Resources Observation Systems (EROS),
Sioux Falls,
South Dakota. 57198,
USA.
Tel: (1) 605 594 6151.
Fax: 605 594 6589

GIFAP (International Group of National Associations of Agrochemical Products).
Avenue Albert,
Lancaster 79A
1180 Bruxelles
Belgium.
Tel: (32) 02 375 6860
Fax; (32) 02 375 2793
Telex: 62120 GIFAP b
This organisation provides booklets, posters and training guides promoting safe use of insecticides. List of publications available on request.

Intermediate Technology Publications
103-105 Southampton Row
London WC1B 4HH
Tel: 071 724 9306
This is the publishing section of the Intermediate Technology Development Group, an organisation which is committed to providing low-cost intermediate technology which will enable poor people in developing countries to take more control of their lives and improve their situation. List of publications available on request.

International Committee of the Red Cross
19, Avenue de la Paix
CH-1202
Geneva,
Switzerland
Tel: (41) 22 346 001
Fax: (41) 22 332 057
This organisation has experience in treating stored relief foods against infestation by storage pests. They also have experience in public health use of insecticides in POW camps and prisons.

International Pesticide Application Research Centre (IPARC)
Silwood Park,
Ascot, Berkshire,
SL5 7PY
UK
Tel: (44) 344 294 234
Fax: (44) 344 294 450
This centre runs courses in pest management and application technology. It collaborates with WHO and can provide information and expertise on insecticide application technology.

Liverpool School of Tropical Medicine
Pembroke Place,
Liverpool L3 5QA
UK
Tel: (44) 51 708 9393
Fax: (44) 51 708 8733
Division of Parasite and Vector Biology has expertise in the biology and

control of a range of disease vectors. The International Health Division runs courses suitable for relief workers. The ODA funded Malaria Consortium is jointly based here and at the London School and provides access to international expertise on malaria control. Runs travel clinic

London School of Hygiene and Tropical Medicine
Keppel Street,
London WCEI 7HT
UK
Tel: (44) 71 636 8636
Fax: (44) 71 636 5389
Department of Medical Parasitology has expertise in the biology and control of a range of disease vectors.
The ODA funded Malaria Consortium is jointly based here and at the Liverpool School and provides access to international expertise on malaria control. MASTA (Medical Advisory Service for Travellers) can provide sachets of permethrin for treating individual nets.

Medical Entomology Centre
at the University of Cambridge
Cambridge Road,
Fulbourne
Cambridge CB1 5EL
Tel: (44) 223 414 316
Fax: (44) 223 416 171
This centre is particularly interested in lice control and runs short courses.

Natural Resources Institute (NRI)
Central Avenue, Chatham, Maritime,
Chatham,
Kent ME4 4TB,
UK.
Tel: (44) 634 880 088
This institute has expertise in the biology and control of some insect vectors/pests (especially tsetse and locust control) and crop/storage pests.
Publications Distribution Office
as above.

United Nations High Commissioner for Refugees.
(UNHCR Technical Support Services)
Palais des Nations
P.O. Box 2500
CH-1211
Geneva 2 D)pot
Switzerland.
Tel: (41) 22 739 8111
Fax: (41) 22 731 9546
This organisations coordinates relief work in refugee camps and may be responsible for compiling guidelines for public health delivery. The local office should always be consulted prior to undertaking a programme. They may have access to relevant unpublished reports from other refugee situations.

World Health Organisation (WHO)
1211 Geneva 27,
Switzerland,
Tel: (41) 22 791 2111
Fax: (41) 22 791 0746
Telex: 415416OMS
WHO support a number of vector control programmes, such as the Onchocerciasis Control Programme and a number of insecticide impregnated bednet programmes. Details of these programmes and unpublished documents concerning vector control and pesticide use can be obtained from:

Control of Tropical Diseases (CTD)
As above.

Official publications and catalogue can be obtained from:
WHO distribution and Sales Unit
Tel: (41) 22 792 2476
Fax: (41) 22 788 0481

WHO catalogue and publications can also be obtained via:
HMSO Publications Centre
51 Nine Elms Lane
London
SW8 5DR
Tel: (44) 71 873 8372

Appendix 2
Addresses of commercial companies

The mention of specific companies or of certain manufacturers' products does not mean that they are endorsed or recommended by the author in preference to others of a similar nature that are not mentioned. The Pesticide Index contains an extensive list of chemical companies. Addresses of other useful companies may be obtained from WHO or IPARC. Try to get as much advice as possible from experienced people.

Cholinesterase test kit
Test-mate OP cholinesterase Kit (includes Test-mate OP analyzer, with battery, instruction manual, breakable field case, all accessary items and Erythrocyte reagent) costs $935 and can be obtained from:
EQM Research Inc.
2585 Montana Ave.
Cincinnati,
OH 45211
USA
Tel: (1) 513 661 0560
FaxFax: (1) 513 661 0567

Manufacturers of insecticides
The 'off patent' insecticides (such as DDT, and malathion) are now usually made by insecticide manufactures in underdeveloped countries. All the modern insecticides (such as the pyrethroids) are usually patented and often restricted to one or two major manufacturing companies. Insecticides of the same name may have been formulated differently by different manufacturers.

Remember that just because a product is available it does not mean it can be used in every country. National registration regulations should be investigated first. It helps to use companies which have a local agent in the country of use who should assist in getting the registration information.

Table 23 manufacturers of common public health insecticides

Insecticides (Tradenames in *italics*)	Manufacturing company
Mosbar – permethrin treated soap-bar	Simmons Pty LTD, P.O. Box 10-7 Victoria, Australia.
Altosid Methoprene *Teknar* Bacillus thuringiensis H-14	Sandoz Products, Ltd, Lichtstrasse, 35CH-4002, Basle, Switzerland. Tel: (41) 61 324 1111
Skeetal Bacillus thuringienesis H-14	Microbial Resources Inc. 507 ,Lambark Place, Newark, DE 19711 USA Tel: (1) 302 737 4297
Deet	Pfizer Chemicals Europe and Africa, 10 Dover Rd, Kent CT13 OBN, UK. Tel: (44) 304 616 161. Fax: (44) 304 616 221 Telex: 966555.
Perigel Permethrin *K-Othrin* Deltamethrin	Rousel Uclef, Ravens Lane, Berkhamstead, Herts. HP4 2DY, UK Tel: (44) 442 863 333 Fax: (44) 442 872 783
Icon Lamdacylohalythin *Actellic* Pirimiphos methyl	Zeneca Public Health, Fernhurst, Haslemere, Surrey GU 27 3JE. UK Tel: (44) 428 655 329/655 081 Fax: (44) 428 657 080/657 179
Abate Temephos *Malatol* Malathion	American Cyanamid Co., Agricultural Division, 1 Cyanamid Plaza, Wayne, NJ 07470. USA Tel: (1) 201 831 2000.
Baygon Propoxur	Bayer AG. Pflanzenschutzentrum Monheim, 5090 Leverkusen Bayerwerk, Germany Tel: (49) 214 45011
Sumithion Fenitrothion *Sumithrin* d-Phenothrin	Sumitomo Chemical Company Ltd., 15 5-chome Kitahama Higashi-ku Osaka. Tel: (81) 6 220 3745 Fax: (81) 6 220 3745
Ficam Bendiocarb	FMC Agricultural Chemical Group, 2000 Market Street, Philadelphia, PA 19103 USA Tel. (1) 215 299 6565.

Table 24 Manufacturers of common spray machines used in public health

CP3
Knapsack
Hand operated
Continuously pumped

Weight: 6.24 kg
Tank capacity: 18 litres
Polypropylene container

Residual spraying of
surfaces and larviciding

Cooper Pegler & Co Ltd
Burgess Hill
Sussex England, UK
Tel: (44) 444 242 526
Fax: (44) 444 235 578

Fontan **R12**
Knapsack
Power operated
Mist blower

Weight:13.4 kg
Tank capacity: 10 litres
Engine: JL0 2-stroke 60 c.c.
Recoil starter
Performance: Mist carries
10 m vertically; 12 m
horizontally in still air.
Also ULV spraying
attachment optional extra

Space spraying outdoors or
in store rooms Larviciding
large expanses of water

Jaydon Engr.Co.Ltd
258 Sutton Common Rd.
Sutton, Surrey
SM3 9PW
UK
Tel: (44) 81 064 1991

Hudson X-pert
Knapsack
Hand operated
Pressurised

Tank capacity: 14 litres
Stainless steel tank

Residual spraying of
surfaces and larviciding

H.D. Hudson Mfg Co.
Shawnee Mission
Kansas, 66201,
USA
Tel: (1) 913 362 4000

Allman **L80**
Knapsack
Power operated
Mist blower

Weight: 21 kg
Tank capacity: 14 litres
Engine: C7 2-stroke, 77
c.c.
Rope start (recoil starter
extra)

Space Spraying
outdoors or in
storerooms
Larviciding
large expanses
of water

E. Allman & Co Ltd
Birdham Road
Chichester, Sussex
UK
Tel: (44) 243 512 511

Turbair Fox
Rotary atomiser
Hand held
Power operated
Mist blower

Weight: 5 kg
Tank capacity: 1 litre
Engine: 2-stroke
1 h.p.
Standard plastic bottle of
insecticide becomes a tank
by screwing on to sprayer

Space spraying
outdoors or in store rooms

Turbair Ltd
Britannica House
Waltham Cross
Herts.
Tel: (44) 992-623 691

LECO H.D.
Vehicle mounted in Land
Rover or similar vehicle
Power operated
ULV aerosol/fog
generator

Weight: 215 kg
Tank capacity: 44 litres
Engine fuel: Petrol
Air output: 6.08 m /sec
Tank capacity: 52 litres

Produces dense fog for
outdoor or indoor control
of flies and mosquitoes

Rousel Uclef, Ravens
Lane, Berkhamstead,
Herts. HP4 2DY, UK
Tel: (44) 442 863 333
Fax: (44) 442 872 783

Swingfog SN11
Hand held
Power operated
Pulse jet Weight: 9 kg

Tank capacity: 4.5 litres
Operates on pulse jet
principle
Ignition powered by
flashlight batteries

Optional extra, 14 litre
back pack tank for
extended use
Output:10-30 litres/hr
Suitable for oil or
water-based solutions
Carries 20-30 ft in still air

Produces dense fog
Outdoor or indoor
control of flies
and mosquitoes

Jaydon Engr. Co.Ltd.
258 Sutton Common Rd.
Sutton, Surrey.
SM3 9PW
Tel: (44) 81 641 1991

bis Products
4 Node Court
Codicote
Hertfordshire
SG4 8TR
*Supply permethrin-treated
bednets to camping shops.*

LifeSystems
PO Box 1407
London SW3 6PL

*Supply permethrin-treated
bednets to camping shops.*

Appendix 3
Identification of mosquitoes

Diagrammatic representation of the principal characters separating the various stages in the lifecycles of anopheline and culicine mosquitoes

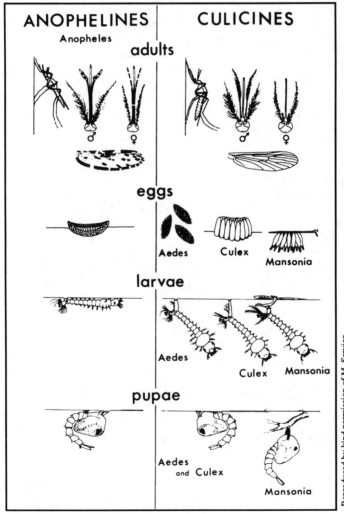

References

Vector-borne diseases and refugee health

There are numerous texts which may be useful. Below are listed a number of recommended texts covering a range of relevant topics.

Appleton (1987) *Drought Relief in Ethiopia: Planning and Management of Feeding Programmes. A Practical Guide,* Save the Children Fund (UK). 186pp.

Benenson, A S (ed) (1990) *Communicable Diseases,* 15th Edition, A report of the American Public Health Association, Washington.

Bres, P (1986) *Public Health Action in Emergencies Caused by Epidemics,* WHO Geneva. 287pp.

Describes a systematic approach to the organisation of an emergency health service, field investigations, analysis of the results and implementation and evaluation of control measures.

Cairncross, S, and Feacham, R (1993) *Environmental Health Engineering in the Tropics: An Introductory Text,* 2nd edition, John Wiley & Sons, Chichester.

Extensively revised and updated from its 1983 edition. Gives details of environmental interventions which will be effective against disease vectors. Essential reading for relief workers in charge of water and sanitation.

Curtis, C (ed.) (1991) *Control of Disease Vectors in the Community,* Wolfe. 233pp.

Gives a well-referenced summary of the state of the art in appropriate vector control technology.

Matthews, G A (1992) *Pesticide Application Methods,* 2nd edition, Longman.

A guide to the theory and practice of pesticide application in agriculture, but highly relevant to vector control.

Meecham, A P (1984) *Rats and Mice, their Biology and Control,* The Rentokil Library. 383pp.

Still the industry's standard textbook on rat and mice control.

Meek, S (1989) 'Vector-borne diseases among displaced Kampucheans', in *Demography and Vector-borne Diseases* (ed. Service, M) CRC Press.

Phillips, M, Mills, A, and Dye, C (1993) *Guidelines for Cost-effectiveness Analysis of Vector Control*, PEEM Guidelines series No. 3. 192pp.
Introduction to cost-effectiveness analysis.

Ramchandran, C P (1993) Control of Lymphatic Filariasis and Onchocrciasis, CTD/MIP/WP.93.5

Service, M (1986) *Lecture Notes on Medical Entomology*, Blackwells, Oxford. 265pp.

Simmonds, S, Vaughan, P, and Gunn, S W, (1983) *Refugee Community Health Care*, Oxford Medical Publication. 357pp.
Major text on refugee health care.

Wisner, B (in prep) A practical guide to environmental health management in disasters and emergencies.
Soon to be published by WHO.

Journal articles

Articles relating to vector-borne disease problems, their treatment and control are widely disseminated in academic journals. Abstracts of these articles can be searched for in many major medical and scientific libraries using the CD-ROM bibliographic programmes such as MEDLINE, POPLINE, LIFE_SCI. These abstracts, which often give a lot of detail, include the name and address of the authors and provide an excellent first insight into who is doing what, and where, in the field of interest. Some relevant papers are listed below.

Brown A E, Meek S R, Maneechai N, Lewis G E (1988) 'Murine typhus among Khmers living at an evacuation site on the Thai-Kampuchean border' *American Journal of Tropical Medicine and Hygiene* 38, 168-171.

Brown, V, Larouze, B, Desve, G, Rousset, J J, Thibon, M, Fourrier, A, and Schwoebel, V (1988) 'Clinical presentation of louse-borne relapsing fever among Ethiopian refugees in northern Somalia' *Annals of Tropical Medicine and Parasitology* 82, 499-502.

Cutts F (1985) 'Community participation in Afghan refugee camps in Pakistan' *Journal of Tropical Medicine and Hygiene* 88, 407-413.

Dick B and Simmonds S (1985) 'Primary health care with refugees: between the idea and the reality' *Tropical Doctor* 15, 2-7.

Henderson P L, and Biellik R J (1983) 'Comparative nutrition and health services for victims of drought and hostilities in the Ogaden: Somalia and Ethiopia, 1980-1981' *International Journal of Health Services* 13, 289-306.

Lindsay, S W and Janneh, L M (1989) 'Preliminary field trials of personal protection against mosquitoes in The Gambia using deet or permethrin in soap, compared with other methods', *Medical and Veterinary Entomology* 3, 97-100.

Rowland, M, Hewitt, S and Durrani, N (1984) 'Prevalence of malaria in Afghan refugee villages in Pakistan sprayed with lamdacyhalothrin or malathion' *Transactions of the Royal Society of Tropical Medicine*, 88, 378-379.

Shears P and Lusty T (1987) 'Communicable disease epidemiology following migration: studies from the African famine' *International Migration Review* 21, 783-795.

Simmonds S P (1984) 'Refugees, health and development' *Transactions of the Royal Society of Tropical Medicine and Hygiene* 78, 726-733.

Stephenson (1981) 'Sanitation and medical care in refugee camps' *Disasters* Vol. 5. No. 3. 281-287.

Thornhill, E W (1984) 'Maintenance and repair of spraying equipment' *Tropical Pest Management* 30, 266-281.

Thornhill, E W (1985) 'A guide to knapsack sprayer selection' *Tropical Pest Management*. 31.

Yip and Sharp (1993) 'Acute malnutrition and high childhood mortality related to diarrhoea: lessons from the 1991 Kurdish refugee crisis', *Journal of the American Medical Association* 170; 587-90.

WHO, (1992) 'Famine-affected refugee and displaced populations: recommendations for public health issues' *Morbidity and Mortality Weekly Report* 24 RR-13 1-76

Available from CTD/WHO

WHO (1982) *Vector Control Series: Lice*. WHO/VBC/82.858. 10pp.

WHO (1982) *Vector Control Series: Cockroaches* WHO/VBC/82.856. 53pp.

WHO (1985) *Vector Control Series: Bed Bugs* VBC/TS.85.2. 26pp.

WHO (1985) *Vector Control Series: Fleas* VBC/TS/85.1. 55pp.

WHO (1986) *Vector Control Series: The Housefly* WHO/VBC/86.937. 63pp.

WHO (1985) *Vector Control Series: Lice* VBC/TS/85.3. 35pp.

WHO (1988) *Vector Control Series: Tsetse Flies* WHO/VBC/88.958. 88pp.

WHO (1987) *Vector Control Series: Rodents* WHO/VBC/87.949. 107pp.

The documents in Vector Control Series are divided into 'advanced' and 'middle' level training guides. The former is aimed at MSc. level professional staff while the latter is aimed at less specialised community workers.

WHO (1988) *The WHO Recommended Classification of Pesticides by Hazard and Guidelines to Classification 1988-1989* WHO/VBC/88.953. 39pp.

WHO (1983) *Methods of Disposal of Surplus Pesticides and Pesticide Containers in Developing Countries* WHO/VBC/83.884 10pp.

Other valuable unpublished texts may be available from CTD.

Available from publications office/WHO or nearest WHO agent

Publications catalogue: 1986-90, 1991, 1992, 1993. As well as the list of new books published (including English language books of PAHO after 1990) this catalogue lists the major distributers in countries around the world. Publications may have been translated into a number of languages.

WHO (1992) *Entomological Field Techniques for Malaria Control. Part I. Learners Guide* WHO Nonserial publication. 77pp.

WHO (1992) *Entomological field techniques for Malaria Control Part II Tutor's Guide* WHO Nonserial publication. 54pp.

These two field manuals are ideal for use in training staff involved in a malaria control programme

WHO (1989) *Geographical Distribution of Arthropod-borne Diseases and their Principal Vectors* WHO/VBC/89.967.

This manual provides information on the geographical distribution of the main diseases transmitted by mosquitoes, ticks, mites, lice, tsetse flies, cone-nosed (kissing) bugs, phlebotomine sandflies, fleas, blackflies, and deer flies. In addition the distribution of the most important vectors is described in short texts, illustrated with over 100 maps.

Technical Report Series. International groups of experts summarise world knowledge on a given disease.

WHO (1986) *Expert Committee on Malaria. 18th Report.* WHO Tech. Rep. Ser. 735:, 104pp.

WHO (1985) *Arthropod-Borne and Rodent-Borne Viral Diseases.* Tech. Rep. Ser. No.719. 116pp.

WHO (1992) *Lymphatic Filariasis: The Disease and its Control. Fifth report of the WHO expert committee on filariasis.* Tech. Rep. Ser. No. 821. 71pp.

WHO (1980) *Environmental Management for Vector Control.* Tech. Rep. Ser. A/2/80. 75pp.

WHO (1992) *Vector Resistance to Pesticides. Fifteenth report of the WHO expert committee on vector biology and control.* Tech. Rep. Ser. 818. 62pp.

WHO (1987) *Vector Control in Primary Health Care.* Tech. Rep. Ser. No.755. 61pp.

Offset manuscripts and non serial publications

WHO (1972) *Vector Control in International Health.* Nonserial Publication. 144pp.

Particularly useful for identifying different vectors/pests and with excellent section on rodent control

WHO (1982) *Manual on Environmental Management for Mosquito Control: With Special Emphasis on Malaria Vectors.* WHO Offset Publication No.66. 283pp.

WHO (1973) *Manual on Larval Control Operations in Malaria Programmes.* WHO Offset Publication No.1. 199pp.

WHO (1989) *The Use of Impregnated Bednets and Other Materials for Vector-borne Disease Control* (WHO/VBC/89.981).

This booklet provides a comprehensive summary of pre 1989 bednet trials and gives advice on operational management and socio-economic aspects of a net-impregnation programme.

WHO (1993) *Equipment for Vector Control* (3rd Edition). WHO Nonserial Publication. 310pp.

An illustrated guide to the technical design, calibration, performance, safe use, maintenance and testing of virtually all equipment, from hand operated sprayers to fixed-wing aircraft.

WHO (1991) *Insect and Rodent Control Through Environmental Management: A Community Action Programme.* WHO Nonserial kit

Contains book, cards, games. 107.

PAHO (1982) *Emergency Vector Control after Natural Disaster.* PAHO Scientific Publication No.419. 98pp.

Available from UNHCR

UNHCR (1982) *Handbook for Emergencies.* 194pp

UNHCR (1989) *Guidelines for Environmental Health Services for Afghan Refugees in Pakistan.* 75pp.

UNHCR (1988) *Manual for Operation and Maintenance of the Hudson Sprayer.* 25pp

UNHCR (unpublished) A Framework for People-orientated Planning in Refugee Situations: Taking Account of Women, Men, and Children.

Walsh J F (1982) 'Enquiry into the transmission of onchocerciasis in the proposed refugee resettlement area of the Poli Arrondissement (NorthCameroon) with suggestions on the siting of villages' (unpublished report to the UNHCR.)

Available from GIFAP

Many of these publications are available in French, English and Italian.

Booklets

GIFAP (1984) *Guidelines for Emergency Measures in Cases of Pesticide Poisoning.* 49pp.
GIFAP (1983) *Guidelines the Safe and Effective Use of Pesticides.* 58pp.
GIFAP (1987) *Guidelines for the Safe Transport of Pesticides.* 62pp.
GIFAP (1989) *Guidelines for Personal Protection when Using Pesticides in Hot Climates.* 34pp.
GIFAP (1987) *Guidelines for the Avoidance, Limitation and Disposal of Pesticide Waste on the Farm.* 44pp.

Posters

GIFAP (1983) Guidelines for the safe and effective use of pesticides
GIFAP (1984) Guidelines for emergency measures in case of pesticide poisoning

Slides are also available.

Available from NRI

NRI (1990) Natural Resistance of 85 West African Hardwood Timbers to Attack by Termites and Micro-organisms
Kidd, H, and James, J R (1994) Pesticide Index 282pp.
  This valuable reference list of pesticide names and manufactures is available free of charge to non-profit making organisations in countries eligible for British Government Aid.

Available from Intermediate Technology Publications

Technical briefs (four pages long, relying heavily on diagrams; each brief ends with an indication of where to go for more information).
An Introduction to Pit Latrines (no. 2)
Choosing a Water-seal Latrine (No. 6)
Making Soap (No. 8)
Health, Water, and Sanitation (No. 17)
Public and Communal Latrines (No. 28)
Latrine Vent Pipes (No. 32)

These notes have been collected together, and published, with additional material, in the following manual:

IT (1991) *The Worth of Water: Technical Briefs on Health, Water and Sanitation* (32pp)

Index